Yoga for Back Pain Relief

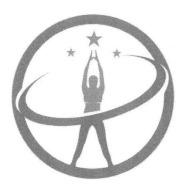

by Julia Meadows

About the Author

Julia Meadows is a senior coach at Mindset Mastership, a life coaching business based in London, England.

Mindset Mastership teaches clients how human behavior really works. Through our teaching, we have helped clients worldwide gain a better advantage, to develop themselves and achieve more from life.

For further details, see:

MindsetMastership.com

Want free goodies?

Email us at:

mindsetmastership@gmail.com

Find us on Instagram!

@MindsetMastership

Most people have no idea just how their body & mind has been designed to feel good.

Table of Contents

Introduction 1

About this Book.. 3

Chapter 1: What is Yoga.. 5

Importance of Yoga 6

Yoga in Our Daily Life 7

Yoga Is a Great Stress Buster 8

Yoga Promotes Whole-Body Fitness......................9

When to Practice 10

Where to Practice 11

Eating and Drinking................................ 12

What to Wear...................................... 12

What You Need..................................... 12

Chapter 2: Muscle Balance in Yoga 13

What is a muscle imbalance? 16

Does Traditional Yoga Lead to Muscular Imbalance? 16

The Shoulder Strength Imbalance in Yoga 17

Chapter 3: Side Effects of Yoga 23

Positive Side Effects 24

Possible Negative Side Effects........................ 25

Chapter 4: How Yoga Helps with Pain Management 29

How Pain Affects our Brain.........................30

How Does Yoga Actually Help Us Process and Perceive Pain?
.... 31

How asanas fight pain 32

In what ways pranayama helps to relax our body and
anxieties... 32

Common Pain Conditions and How Yoga Helps 34

Emotional Healing Yoga Poses 36

Spiritual Meanings of Yoga Postures 48

Psychic Development 54

Chapter 5: Yoga and Pain 57

Yoga and pain 58

What is the evidence for yoga's effectiveness when you have
pain? 59

How to choose a Yoga teacher and class? 60

Can anyone do yoga? 60

Can I do yoga at home? 60

Do I need to tell my health care professional I am doing yoga?
.... 61

All about pain 61

THE PROTECTIVE PAIN RESPONSE 62

UNDERSTANDING CHRONIC PAIN 63

PAIN AGAIN 64

UNLEARNING PAIN THROUGH RELAXATION 65

BREATHING THE WHOLE BODY 66

A RESTORATIVE YOGA ROUTINE FOR CHRONIC PAIN.68

NESTING POSE 69

SUPPORTED BOUND ANGLE POSE.. 70

SUPPORTED BACKBEND POSE... 70

**Chapter 6: Beginners Exercises to Heal Back-Pain
Scoliosis at Home 73**

Stretches and exercises for scoliosis 74

9 Yoga Poses for Upper Back Pain 87

8 stretches for the middle back 98

5 Yoga Poses to Ease Lower Back Pain 114

10 Yoga Poses for Sciatica Pain Relief............................ 120

5 Yoga Poses to Avoid If You Have Piriformis Syndrome... 135

The 4 Best Stretching Exercises to Ease Groin Pain 141

Chapter 7: Soreness After Yoga 147

Hydrate, then hydrate a little more.............................. 149

DO get plenty of sleep... 149

DON'T down caffeine and energy supplements...................... 149

DO exercise—gently.. 149

Use a foam roller 150

DO eat a balanced meal 150

DON'T take anti-inflammatory drugs 150

DO take a hot bath... 150

DO stretch... 151

DON'T do intense stretching.. 151

DO continue to practice yoga, gently 151

Chapter 8: Discover How Yoga Poses and Meditation can Improve Your Anatomy.. 153

38 Ways Yoga Improves Anatomy 154

Chapter 9: How to Meditate 171

Introduction 172

What is meditation? 173

EXAMPLES OF MEDITATION....................................... 174

CATEGORIES OF MEDITATION 174

How to Meditate... 175

CONCENTRATIVE TECHNIQUES 176

Tips for Applying the Concentrative Techniques.............. 176

Positioning.. 177

Quieting the Mind 178

FOCUS ON THE BREATH 179

VARIATIONS ON A THEME 180

Expressing Gratitude.. 181

SETTLING INTO THE MEDITATIVE MOMENT 181

Movement Meditation through Martial Arts 182

EXPRESSIVE MEDICATION: CREATING AN OUTLET FOR MEDITATING 183

Conclusions 184

Chapter 10: How to Use Meditation to Manage Chronic Pain 187

1. The pain is not all in your head 187

2. The paradox of paying attention 188

3. Regulating the response 189

4. Putting the pieces together... 190

Chapter 11: Science-Based Benefits of Meditation.. 193

1. Reduces stress.. 194
2. Controls anxiety.. 195
3. Promotes emotional health 196
4. Enhances self-awareness................................... 197
5. Lengthens attention span 197
6. May reduce age-related memory loss.................. 198
7. Can generate kindness....................................... 199
8. May help fight addictions.................................. 200
9. Improves sleep.. 201
10. Helps control pain 202
11. Can decrease blood pressure............................203
12. You can meditate anywhere..............................204

Chapter 12: Ayurvedic Diet Plan: Get Rid of any Disease with One Diet 207

Ayurvedic Diet Plan...207
Ayurvedic Diet: Meal Timings...............................209
Ayurvedic Diet: Morning Meal............................. 210
Morning Food Ratio 210
Morning Fruits 211
Restricted foods in the Morning 211
Ayurvedic Diet: Evening Meal.............................. 212
Evening Food Ratio 212

Conclusion 213

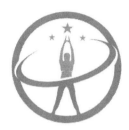

Introduction

Yoga, which includes anything from stretches to meditation, is the most effective overall form of pain reduction ever studied. The explanation is simply because yoga is so effective in controlling stress. Through severe pain, your body's stress response system — such as the sympathetic nervous system and hormones like cortisol — stays stuck in the "on" position. Simply being in a position of "fight or flight" prepares you well for an imminent risk to life or health, but it is generally ineffective when it comes to chronic pain. Upon tension, you appear to breathe quicker and more erratically. Muscles tense. Your mood could crash. This can make the pain worse.

The more and steadier you practice yoga, the greater the improvements in brain and your nervous system wiring. We use the body and breath that we can regulate to some extent to relax, activate, and eventually reinforce the nervous system and the mind that are typically beyond control. As this balances your nervous system and mind, you are ready to respond to whatever problems arise.

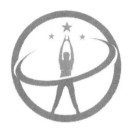

About this Book

This book, **Yoga for Pain Relief,** is different from any of the others out there. Because of the way the book is structured, it is easy to find the answer you are searching for. Go ahead and click through the book and see for yourself. Nice bold headings guide your eyes to just the section you need, and for a fast response, you do not have to read the entire text. This book is a comprehensive overview of all aspects of yoga, from introduction to pain management. You will need information on what to do and how to do yoga. There is detail here too. So put this book in a prominent position on your bookshelf. We are sure you are going to return to it again and again.

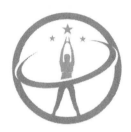

Chapter 1:

What is Yoga

Yoga was founded by an Indian Hindu called Patanjali in the year 300 and the word itself means yoke or union. Yoga as a concept is a balance between spirit, body, and mind. Yoga's theory is to stretch the muscles, stabilize the body, increase focus, relax and, most importantly, provide higher consciousness awareness.

For thousands of years, yoga has been a tradition of the physical and mental health system, initially in India, its source, and now gradually across the globe. One of the characteristics of its success is the fact that even doctors recommend the importance of yoga, and scientists are intensively researching it. In summary, yoga soothes and calms both body and mind, while it elevates the spirit. It is an outstanding discipline to get well and remain well.

Yoga is a collection of techniques that represents scientific principles that are true and tested. Yoga practitioners have long understood many things that Western scientists are coming to appreciate about the body. Yoga views the body from a different viewpoint than that of conventional Western medicine, but the basic concepts are the same. What we Westerners call the nerve plexus, yoga calls chakras. (These words do not necessarily coincide, as chakras contain psychospiritual energy.)

Importance of Yoga

The value of yoga in our lives has been brought to the attention of Western countries, like the United States, after it gained prominence because of its many marketed advantages. Yoga for a better lifestyle and yoga for the elderly have become a common additions in fitness centers across the globe and in personal health schedules, for excellent reasons. The methods of yoga and its wellness benefits are why people have discovered its numerous healing, body, and mind attributes.

The importance of yoga in our lifestyles is already seen from the beginner's point of view on methods of meditation, yoga healing and relaxation, wellbeing and maternity yoga, as well as weight-loss yoga, and other approaches to yoga that are so popular today. Yoga's role in our lives and yoga's health benefits are plentiful, so if you have not tried it yet, go ahead and seek a good old academy.

Yoga in Our Daily Life

Yoga is more a lifestyle or mental state than an activity. The benefits extend well beyond the physical body. You will reap these advantages as long as you are practicing daily.

The benefits of yoga are prompted by the focus on inner harmony. The foundation stones of yoga are self-realization, concentration, relaxation, and harmony. One of the best things about yoga is that there is no charge irrespective of the advantages it provides. There really is no actual training equipment needed to practice yoga, or particular surroundings. The magnificence of yoga is that after the very first session the benefits are apparent. And it does not depend on your level of versatility, or whether you can get into the poses in full.

Yoga benefits are both precautionary and curative. Daily yoga practice makes the body strong from the inside out. When the body is in complete balance, there is a decrease in the risk of sickness. Practicing mornings and evenings can be of great benefit. Practicing morning workouts will lead to a healthy body and mind during the day and improve one's lifestyle. A session also helps induce peaceful and restful sleep.

Yoga Is a Great Stress Buster

Stress is a basic fact of twenty-first-century life on earth; stress is so normal that countries around the globe have integrated the English word "stress" into their own tongues. If you have not been under stress, then we would like to share your secret. (It is actually yoga!) Yoga addresses multiple types of tension. The postures, or asanas, help you regulate your restless body, making it stronger and more flexible, functioning better and, ultimately, more resistant to disease and other physical issues. Asanas practice teaches the body to do exactly what you are asking it to do. Your doctor knows that regular exercise, breathing exercises, and relaxation are all excellent ways of relieving stress — yoga helps out all three.

Breathing exercises in Yoga, or pranayama, actively channel the flow of life energy, or prana, in and out of the body. Physiologically, intense, frequent breathing sends out a signal for relaxation to every cell in your body. Yoga meditation relaxes racing thoughts while the exercises enhance the ability to control your own mind, rather than allowing it to dominate. Yoga is a way of life, physical, mental, and spiritual, that puts life in perspective. Yoga does not change challenging situations, but it does educate you how to respond to them without neglecting or hurting yourself.

Yoga Promotes Whole-Body Fitness

You might be an experienced athlete, or you might be a couch potato looking for the remote control. Why Yoga practice? Three days a week at the gym is fine. Yoga is great for you, too! As yoga incorporates so many different fitness elements and is so easily adapted to the person, it can be practiced both at the beginner and at the most advanced level with equal benefit. If you are a novice or an advanced student, yoga will loosen up your body slowly, gently, and easily. You will feel stronger, breathe better, and move more easily. The idea that yoga is not competitive may not attract you.

In reality, in direct contrast to what is thought to be the yoga frame of mind, a sense of personal competition is part of it. Your practice of yoga is personal and may have little to do with anyone else. But yoga can give you so much strength, and such an enhanced self-image that you find that exercise is not as bad as you think. Yoga is designed to work all the muscles, not just a certain isolated large group. Some of the postures, such as flips and inversions, activate different internal organs, or produce energy from stress-prone areas like the lower back or neck.

Fine-tuning one's program with yoga makes for the perfect complete-body workout. Other workout plans aim to only improve a portion of your body — for example, cardiovascular health, leg strength, or fat burning. Yoga does all of that. While there are many forms, Hatha Yoga is the type of that focuses on the body and is the most emphasized form of in this book and practiced by Westerners. Hatha Yoga is a fantastic fitness system, but it is more. Hatha Yoga is based on the belief that the secret to calming your mind and liberating your spirit is to achieve absolute power over your body.

Heart disease is approximately twice as likely to occur in physically inactive people according to the National Heart, Lung, and Blood Institute. Our society is undergoing increasing movement towards spiritual issues. Despite a growing enthusiasm for holistic approaches to health, we are a society seeking equilibrium in an out-of-control environment. Holistic exercise is fast becoming a common term and yoga fits into this phenomenon comfortably. Yoga is the response to the quest for physical perfection for the spiritual seeker and the athlete, because it is the best all-purpose, all-person, all-self, individualized form of fitness.

When to Practice

Set aside a clear time to enjoy the practice of yoga in your day. Dawn and dusk are regarded as the best times of day, as the rising and lowering of the sun brings unique energy into our bodies. But, if you cannot find these moments, find another time of the day that suits you better, and practice regularly. Practice throughout the morning if you really want to organize your body and mind for the day and bring positive energy into your body first thing.

Practice in the evening after a hard day to relax, unwind, and concentrate. The body should be more relaxed during the evening, and you can go further into more difficult postures.

Where to Practice

Choose a place with the least possible disturbance. It can be your house, garden, the beach - indoors or outdoors, anywhere an even, flat surface is available. Ensure that the room is ventilated and at a reasonable temperature if you work indoors. It is not advisable to have air-conditioned rooms. The body is rigid when cold, and tissues stretch slowly. A healthy atmosphere and fresh air supplement the breathing exercises with added benefits.

Ensure you have enough range to move about freely, stretching your arms and legs. Switch off your phone and place a note on your door to indicate that you are taking time for yourself. It is your turn.

Eating and Drinking

Never exercise straight after eating. You should do yoga on an empty stomach. So, give at least 1 hour after a snack and 2-3 hours after a huge meal before you start your workout. Before or after your session, it is best to drink to prevent dehydration. Prevent drinking water during the session to avoid losing your focus on breathing and the yoga postures. When you train in the morning, however, have at least one glass of hot water before your practice, or a small snack (fruit or yogurt). Have a proper breakfast when you are done with your workout.

What to Wear

Wear comfortable clothes, light and loose, usually made of natural fibers. Your clothing should not limit your movement. If necessary, remove jewelry, your watch and glasses. Yoga is best done with bare feet.

What You Need

Get yourself a special yoga pad. Padding or a non-slip surface makes the work smoother and safer. One can be found at any sports store. Nobody else should use your mat. This is not just for purposes of hygiene, but also because you will eventually produce energy on your mat that will help you during the yoga practice. You can play calming, soothing music in the background, if you like - just make sure it is not too loud.

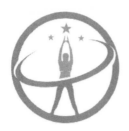

Chapter 2:

Muscle Balance in Yoga

"Yoga is the study of equilibrium, and the goal of all living creatures is balance: it is our place"

In America, one hundred million people suffers from severe pain. Chronic pain is defined as pain that lasts a long time like six months. The number goes even higher when we add acute pain. Severe and chronic pain can be unbearable from mild to severe. Per year, living with pain costs society more than $600 billion. It is a big public health concern. As a neuromuscular consultant, I have found that neck back, knee, and headache pains are the four most common complaints from clients.

In reality, I am going to bet many of you reading this book have suffered from these problems or know someone who has. At any stage in their lives, some people definitely feel acute pain and chronic pain. Interestingly, when some of us were growing up back in the 1950s, low back pain was one of the most common reasons that caused a person to seek medical attention. Low back pain today, in 2020, is still one of the most likely reasons a person seeks medical treatment. Why is it that low back pain is still so common in a country with such an advanced medical system? The reason is that they generally treat symptoms when a doctor or therapist tackles low back pain, and not the cause.

Treating the symptoms to obtain relief is, of course, fine, but treating the source of the low back pain in long term would provide more enduring relief. There is evidence that the root cause of several forms of neuro-muscular pain is seen in the biomechanical misalignments induced by muscle imbalances. Therapists often refer to this as long locked or short locked muscles.

You may be diagnosed with any one of hundred diseases by your doctor. In our Western medicine model, normal care for conditions such as plantar fasciitis, sciatica, tennis elbow, carpal tunnel, most headaches, low back pain and herniated discs includes care of the symptoms, usually with a painkiller or anti-inflammatory drug. The cause is seldom handled in Western medicine. I will now reveal to you a "truth" I became conscious of when my headaches were eventually relieved after a car accident. I use the information to help people reduce or remove their neuro-muscular pain almost daily. The trick is to fix muscle imbalances. In my experience, these imbalances can account for 80 percent of a person's lifetime pain! Fixing muscle imbalances will give you improved posture, more strength, and will remove several painful conditions. Muscle imbalances are most often the reason you encounter many serious illnesses in your life, such as:

- Poor posture
- Fascial restrictions
- Nerve compressions
- Disc abnormalities
- Fibromyalgia
- Heel spur (plantar fasciitis)
- knee pain (medial meniscus injury)
- Sciatica (piriformis syndrome)
- Low back pain (lumbar muscle strain)
- CTS (carpal tunnel syndrome)

- Tennis or golfer's elbow (epicondylitis, lateral or medial)
- TOS (thoracic outlet syndrome)
- Neck pain (cervical muscle strain)
- TMJD (temporomandibular joint disorder)
- Tension headaches and migraines

What is a muscle imbalance?

When muscles are either too long or too short, a muscle imbalance exists. This can cause discomfort and likely even inflammation to the muscle system. The optimum functioning of the musculoskeletal system needs a balance of muscles in terms of strength and duration. If muscles do not have this balance, they are painful and the joint where such imbalances occur is may become compromised. In terms of the joint and/or restricted range of motion, this manifests as discomfort.

Does Traditional Yoga Lead to Muscular Imbalance?

Some people who promote yoga believe in its intrinsic ability to achieve balance in mind, body, and spirit. While yoga is a beautiful and therapeutic activity, one aspect of asana is unexpectedly not very stable. Indeed, it is likely to produce an imbalance that can result in physical injury.

"When we investigate asanas of yoga via the scope of anatomy, we can observe that some shoulder muscles are strengthened significantly by asanas while some are barely improved at all."

The word "balance" incorporates a variety of interests from the spiritual to the mental, and the state of physical equilibrium. But the kind of balance I am mentioning here is the functional muscle strength of the shoulders. While we are often told that yoga is a fully balancing activity for the physical body, if we investigate asanas of yoga through the scope of anatomy, we can observe that some shoulder muscles are greatly improved by asanas while some are barely enhanced at all. This muscle mismatch sets the stage for long-term physical harm and injury.

Fortunately, our bodies are continuously adapting to the loads put on them, so this muscle mismatch is not permanent. But the first step towards moving our shoulders to an optimally stable, balanced state is knowledge and understand the problem.

The Shoulder Strength Imbalance in Yoga

To understand how yoga can produce a muscle imbalance in the body, two opposing anatomical acts must be understood:

shoulder-pulling movements and shoulder-pushing movements.

If you use your arms to force an object away from your body, shoulder-pushing motions happen. Imagine pushing on a heavy door or pushing a vacuum cleaner as you clean up your room. When we conduct shoulder-pushing movements using a large range of muscles, we concentrate on the key actors responsible for the action.

Using the body, as you move an object away from you, the muscles that do much of the work are the pectorals (chest muscles), the anterior deltoids (situated at the front of the shoulders), the triceps (muscles along the rear of the upper arms), and the anterior serratus (comprising from the scapulae to the sides of the rib cage). The comparative involvement of each of these muscles differs, depending on the position of the arms and the movement's relation to gravity. Now you can view these four main muscles as collective muscle "pushing."

Let us take an example of shoulder-pushing movements common to yoga practice. We may not use doors or vacuum cleaners in yoga, but we have a broad surface that we constantly push on: the ground underneath the yoga mats. Plank pose is a good illustration of an asana in which we move our arms away from this board. One helpful way to visualize the movement of the shoulders here is to consider what would happen if you did not work your arms in this position.

Your elbows would bend under your weight and gravity if you go all in with your arms; and it would cause the body to fall to the ground (not an attractive picture!). However, instead of falling to the floor, you press off the floor by strengthening your shoulder-pushing muscles (triceps, anterior deltoids, pecs, and anterior serratus) to keep your arms straight to enable your body to swing over the floor.

Unlike pushing movements, shoulder-pulling motions happen as we draw objects towards ourselves. It is like dragging a stubborn weed out of the ground or pulling aggressively on the leash of your dog as he attempts to capture a squirrel. The key muscles that contract are sometimes called antagonistic (or opposing) muscles to the shoulder-pushing muscles. They include the rhomboids and the posterior deltoids (located on the back of each shoulder), the biceps and brachialis muscles (the muscles that line up the forehead with each upper arm), the middle trapezius (located between the scapulae on the upper back), and the latissimus dorsi (otherwise known as the "lats" — those wide, wide back muscles). Again, the relative functioning of these muscles can vary depending on the angle of the arms and on one's relation to gravity. Find that your total shoulder-pulling muscle category.

"We don't really have the equivalent of the stubborn weed or the enthusiastic dog to pull against in yoga and in our practice, there are absolutely no shoulder-pulling motions open to us."

Do you think any typical yoga movements include shoulder-pulling, based on what we know about shoulder-pushing movements? Note that for a yoga pose to correctly fall into this category, it must require pulling something with your arms toward you. What poses demand this? Can you think of any? If you think this is a tricky question, then you are right — good work! The reality is that, in yoga, no objects are present to pull.

Traditional yoga requires only our bodies, the floor, a yoga mat, and the various ways we support our poses (but not by pulling toward us against resistance). In yoga, we do not really use the comparison of the stubborn weed or the enthusiastic dog as an example of pulling, so in practice, there are absolutely no shoulder-pulling movements. When we have an excess of powerful shoulder-pushing movements with no corresponding shoulder-pulling movements, the normal (or unnatural) outcome is a functional force imbalance.

Just to be sure, in no way is this obvious lack of pulling movement in yoga a failure of the practice or supervision. It is literally because the practice of yoga is done completely on the floor on a yoga mat. Many professionals prefer yoga as their main type of physical exercise because it is a long-term health and wellness activity.

Luckily, there are plenty of ways to return our "yoga shoulders" to true functional equilibrium, and it allows us to stretch our range of movement beyond the limits of conventional yoga. Watch for innovative ideas to fix this shoulder strength imbalance — both off and on the yoga mat!

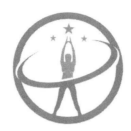

Chapter 3:
Side Effects of Yoga

The success of Yoga is due in large part to the great benefits of daily practice. You can gain peace of mind and improved mental wellbeing, in addition to greater resilience and energy. As in any physical activity, however, some people might even experience adverse side effects. While for most, the positive outweighs the negative, it is necessary to look at all sides of yoga practice.

Positive Side Effects

Exercising only once a week will bring benefits to your mind and body. These involve, but are not limited to, the following:

Muscular strength and flexibility improvement: Even the Disease Control and Prevention Centers mention yoga as a suitable way to fit the prescribed strength-training for perfect health. This side effect of course comes from a muscularly active type of yoga, like vinyasa.

Cardiovascular function improvement: Yoga does not pump your heart as if you were driving a race car or kick boxing, but it has significant cardiovascular side effects that include enhanced strength and stamina, as seen in a study released in the International Journal of Yoga in 2015.

Risk reduction of metabolic disfunction: Yoga will counter some of the causes that put you at risk to metabolic syndrome — an inflammation that produces a greater likelihood of developing heart disease and type 2 diabetes. A 2015 study published in Diabetology and Metabolic Syndrome found that the blood pressure and belly fat of participants with metabolic syndrome were reduced by routine yoga practice for one year.

Enhancement in joint function and flexibility: You eventually get rigid or trapped in particular patterns when you do not shift your joints and muscles in a multitude of directions. Yoga is a type of three-dimensional movement.

Better mental health: Yoga enhances concentration, allays mental fatigue and improves mental health. A 2011 research study published in the International Journal of yoga stated that its practice helps with the reduction of anxiety, addiction, and depression.

Possible Negative Side Effects

Yoga is not just about respirating and calming. It is a very real physical activity with possible adverse side effects. An international study of yoga experts shows that sixty-two percent of those with a musculoskeletal injury found that it lasted more than one month. However, a 2012 broad survey of 2,500 Australian yoga learners reported in the International Yoga Journal revealed that nearly 79 percent of yogis seemed to have no injury at all. Such contrasting findings possibly reflect the type of yoga practice performed. Ashtanga is a physical activity that allows participants to gain hyper-flexibility, which most likely contributed to the occurrence of injury in the above-mentioned report.

Several side effects of yoga are uncommon; in general, the practice is considered healthy. A study of the literature published in the 2013 issue of PLOS ONE recorded only 76 confirmed cases of yoga-related negative side effects:

Complications with glaucoma: Glaucoma is a disease where excess pressure behind the eyeball inevitably contributes to a loss of vision. When you perform some yoga positions, normally inversions like the headstand or shoulder stand, eye pressure rises, causing complications.

Aggravation of high blood pressure: Fast breathing and reversal poses can raise blood pressure, too. When you have pre-existing hypertension, you can be contraindicated to such advanced yoga activities as Breath of Fire.

Back injury: Over-aggressively practiced forward folds can frustrate already vulnerable disks in the back, particularly those in your lumbar spine. Extreme rounding or trying to go too far when you get heated up are forms of serious side effects on the spinal cord.

Muscle strain: In the study PLOS ONE, the muscle system was affected by 27% of reported adverse incidents. This indicates a pull or pressure against a large group of muscles. If you disregard the warning signs of your body and try to expand beyond your established limits, an overstretch can occur. Extend out until you feel a gentle pull, but do not go for intense strain or a drag.

Some populations obviously run a higher risk of suffering adverse side effects from yoga practice. If you have a preexisting medical condition, it is best to check with your personal doctor before attending a session.

Also, it will set you up for injury to train too hard for your level of experience and not to be conscious when you step into certain postures. It is best to work under the guidance of a professional instructor to keep yourself safe from side effects.

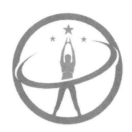

Chapter 4:
How Yoga Helps
with Pain Management

Pain comes at various stages of life, and in many ways. If you have been momentarily dealing with pain or are facing everyday struggles, you know that pain is both a mental and physical battle. The International Association for the Study of Pain (IASP) describes pain as an emotional sensation that is subjective, due to real or possible injury. Do you recognize that definition? Pain is not just a panic response but an emotional reaction. Usually pain perception happens first in our minds and then physiologically.

As per the National Institute of Health (NIH), "Pain is one of the key reasons Americans turn to alternative health strategies such as yoga, meditation and relaxation — which may help relieve pain and other symptoms that are not adequately treated by prescription medications and other traditional therapies." This is because yoga tackles pain both physically and psychologically from either perspective.

Before we delve into the ways yoga can help relieve physical pain, let us think about the mental effects of pain.

How Pain Affects our Brain

Our brain structure is unchanged until our body experiences the actual sense of pain. Chronic pain especially decreases the amount of gray matter in our brain.

Gray matter is the darker brain tissue containing nerve cell bodies as its shelter. The volume and size of the gray matter tissue relates to one's pain tolerance according to (NIH) - the acronym of National Institutes of Health. The greyer matter with pain control will be better. Studies have shown that continued yoga practice contributes to a rise in gray matter in the brain. As the result of age, the amount of gray matter has been shown to decline. The detrimental effects of chronic brain pain can be counteracted by yoga. In other cases, physical pain is the culprit. This is the product of prolonged intense muscle stress, which has an adverse effect on microcirculation. A sedentary lifestyle, lack of exercise, and poor posture will further aggravate the discomfort one feels from pain.

How Does Yoga Actually Help Us Process and Perceive Pain?

Yoga not only changes our brain's internal anatomy, but it also influences how we deal with pain anticipation. This refers to our nervous system. It's because the pranayama (breathing exercises) and asanas (yoga poses) performed in tandem during yoga work to relieve tension and activate the relaxation response of the body. This counteracts the negative effects on the stress response known as "fight or flight." Dr Herbert Benson, the creator of Harvard's Mind and Body Medical School, coined the word "relaxation response". This response to relaxation consists of slow breathing, a reduction in blood pressure and metabolic rate and a decrease in muscle tension. Research suggests that daily yoga practice and mindful meditation build a reflex action that can more easily deliver a sense of calm over time.

But the benefits of yoga go far further than catalyzing the body's reaction to relaxation. Yoga's physical aspects are intended to improve energy, endurance, and flexibility, while mindfulness and meditation are intended to help practitioners gain greater knowledge of their bodies and relieve anxiety.

How asanas fight pain

Asanas muscular stretches improve the working of the body, increase blood flow, correct posture, readjust our skeletal system and improve our muscles. Tandem contractions, with spinal movements and an increased sense of control over one's own body, help alleviate pain.

In what ways pranayama helps to relax our body and anxieties

Feeling pain also affects the intensity and frequency of breathing patterns for two reasons. One is psychological, while the other has to do with the learned habit of slowly "immobilizing" the area to prevent further damage. Breathing may become limited if this area is in the torso. Breathing also becomes slow and forced when one is in pain. The autonomic nervous system has two branches that controls involuntary body functions like the parasympathetic nervous and sympathetic nervous systems. When most people experience pain, it causes the sympathetic nervous system's "fight-or-flight" response, which also involves triggering skyrocketing cortisol levels and forced breathing.

On the other side of the coin, studies show that when yogis fear pain, it activates the parasympathetic nervous system. This provides an answer to the concepts of "tend-and-befriend" or "rest-and-digest," as opposed to the to "fight-or-flight" response. Even though there is less discussion about the emotional experience of pain, the effects of yoga are massive. While yoga is most widely known for helping with physical pain control, there are significant benefits in relaxing the mind during pain. The breathing techniques that yogis perform help them better deal with stressful circumstances, in a situation of anxiety or an actual pain experience.

Pranayama is a systematic method of breath-control. These deep breathing exercises in yoga are known to calm the muscles of the body and reduce nervous thoughts. Some research indicates that pranayama reduces central nervous system activity to calm us down. Breathing exercises that help to relieve anxiety are particularly relevant for pain patients who experience increasing fear of their situation. Such individuals are afraid that physical activity will only intensify their discomfort. This is not always the case, as long as it is done attentively. To sum up, yoga is useful in the treatment of musculoskeletal issues, such as relieving discomfort from inflammation and tight muscles while increasing the release of endorphins that alleviate pain. However, if it is poorly done, it may encourage chronic pain issues.

Common Pain Conditions and How Yoga Helps

#1. Chronic low back pain

Back pain arises from imbalances and the improper positioning of the musculoskeletal elements in the back. Whether it is an injury that causes back pain, sleeping on a bad sleeping surface, obesity or a genetic condition, yoga practice may act as a natural pain reliever. This is because different asanas followed by stretches increase tension in the core muscles for stabilization, which is essential for a healthy back. It is also assumed that yoga helps pain patients gain further trust of physical activity during rising movements (instead of the fear it will make it even worse). The implementation of certain yoga poses gradually by individuals with low back pain is significant. The initiation too early on of strengthening asanas will make the pain worse.

#2. Arthritis

Recent research findings, according to the Arthritis Foundation, indicate that when people with various forms of arthritis frequently practice yoga, it can help alleviate joint pain, increase strength, and functioning in the joints, while relieving stress and tension. In certain cases, asanas need to be changed for patients with arthritis but this is certainly a choice for those dealing with the disease.

#3. Fibromyalgia

Fibromyalgia is a chronic pain condition defined manifested in discomfort and extreme sensitivity to touch throughout the entire body. Fibromyalgia affects more than 10 million Americans, 80 percent being women. Individuals dealing with this condition have a very low pain tolerance.

Fibromyalgia is not healed by it, but yoga will help moderate the condition. The yoga-catalyzed relaxation response poses and deep breathing exercises help alleviate muscle stress and boost attitude.

#4. Migraines

More than 38 million people in the United States experience migraines. It is normal to associate these chronic headaches with stress. Preliminary tests of yoga as a migraine treatment show promising results. In addition to stretches facilitating full body relaxation, yogic breathing also helps stabilize the nervous system and relieve stress.

Emotional Healing Yoga Poses

Yoga soothes suffering and lightens painful memories. By extricating the practitioner from the real pain and by concentrating on optimistic feelings and memories, one learns to deal with pain. Yoga is a traditional practice that does not restrict the lifestyle of an individual in relationship to body movement. Every human has five interconnected layers:

- Annamaya kosha (made from food)
- Pranamaya kosha (the prana)
- Manomaya kosha (the mind and feelings)
- Vijnanamaya kosha (Intelligence, sagacity)
- Anandamaya kosha (bliss, joy)

Any mental distress shows up as illness. Yet one can relieve the mental distress and suffering through prana and yoga. The heart can be opened with back flexion, and one can alleviate symptoms with forward folds, as per the yoga community.

The pelvic area is correlated with the second or Sacral Chakra that is regarded as the storeroom of blocked emotional responses. The spine is implied in the world of our emotions and each cell emits the energy of the composite of mind, body, and strength of character. A healthful body has a frequency between 62–68 Hz. A malignant body has 42 Hz and much less capacity. Good thoughts can boost energy by 10 Hz and bad thoughts by minus 12 Hz.

Pigeon Pose

Pigeon pose or Eka Pada Rajakapotasana is believed to be a hips opener that removes muscular tension all across the pelvic region. Blocked thoughts make their way into the hip.

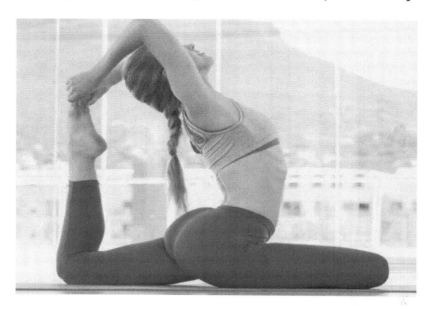

Instructions

- Lie on your knees and palms and begin on all fours.
- Move the right arm in and out.
- Then push the left knee directly backwards. The leg location should appear identical to the design of an L.
- This posture can be achieved from the downward dog stance or from the lung one too.
- Place your hands on the ground next to you, extend your spinal column and push your torso forward, so

that your arms are straight and your head touches the ground or mat. Your abdomen lies over the right hip.

- The stress on both of the knees must be maintained evenly and the knee must suffer no pressure.
- Continue on for five breaths or relax as you are.
- Finally lift the body with the aid of your arms and return to your hands and knees or to the lower side dog stance.

Bow Pose

Bow Posture is a back turn, or Dhanurasana. Back bends support opening the heart and making pain free. It removes tension and tiredness.

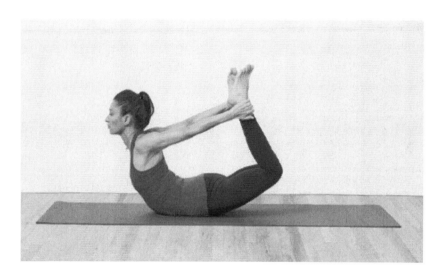

Instructions

- Lie with your arms at the side of your chest. Hold feet hips-width apart.
- Cross the arms and try your best to protect the ankles.
- When you breathe, lift your shoulders and your legs upward from the ground immediately as far as you can.
- Just stare straight ahead and take deep breaths for about 20 seconds.

- Slowly return the legs and body down on the floor as you exhale.
- Loosen the ankles in the initial position.

Seated Forward Bend

Forward bends allow one to concede on pushing higher or removing the unnoticed. It assists in disassociating from the experience.

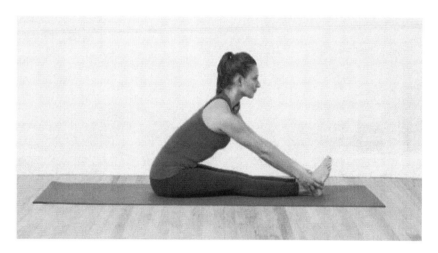

Instructions

- Lie down right in with legs extended. The vertebrae will be upright.
- Lift your hands above your head as you inhale.
- Move the hip joints forward, pulling the knees forward to meet the feet. The backbone remains upright.
- Relax your hands on your legs, extend your backbone and grab your toes. Pull the chin to the knees and aim to imagine the legs as lean as possible.
- Straighten to a sitting posture after around twenty seconds and bend your shoulders.

Sitting Half Spinal Twist

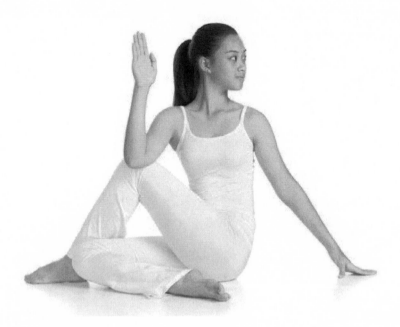

The spine is the infrastructure of the nerves that holds memories. You are activating the spine even you are sitting, laying, or standing, altering one's perceptions. It opens the heart too.

Instructions

- Sit down right with the legs spread with toes together. The backbone should be upright.
- Raise the left leg so that the opposite foot sole lies on the floor away from the right hip as well as the left ankle. Conversely you should hold your left leg straight.

- Move your right knee and push it over your left hip. The positioning of each of the legs will seem like a triangle.
- Put your right hand behind you and your left hand on your right knee to stabilize your body position.
- Bend the knees sideways, as well as the shoulders and the neck, to allow the heel of the bent leg to touch the other as illustrated. Bend to the right.
- Keep your back straight and take long, soft breaths.
- Release the position and rest.
- Repeat instructions on the opposite side.

Malasana

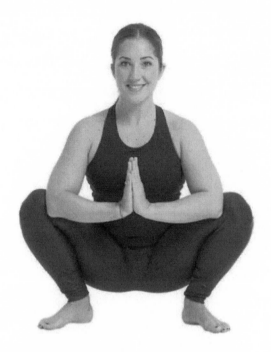

The garland pose is a deep, broad-footed squat that is also a hip opener.

Instructions

- Get as near as feasible into the squat position with bent knees. The feet will rest upon the floor.
- Expand your hips more than the size of your torso.
- In anjali mudra, bend forward and place your elbows across your inner knees.

Shavasana

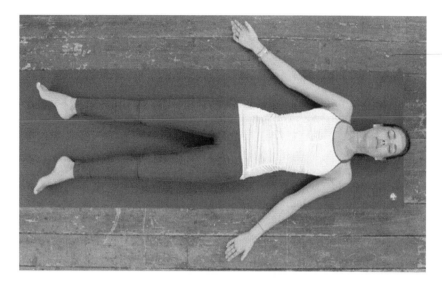

Corpse pose assists in distracting the body from negative opinions and pain that emanate from corporal damage, a broken heart, failed relationships, and/or abusive behavior. In this posture, focus is on various areas of the body one at a time, and the whole body becomes comfortable.

Instructions

- Lie on your back with the knees slightly apart, arms and hands towards the sky along your body.
- Focus on right foot, then switch to the right knee and from then to the thighs. Do the same with your left leg.
- Push your consciousness slowly up to head across every portion of the body.

- Calm your body and shift your senses from top to bottom and vice versa.
- Move after about twenty minutes for almost one minute.
- Sit patiently in a posture of ease.
- Be conscious of your environment and body after few deeper breaths, and finally open up your eyes.

Yoga doesn't just mean physical activity. It involves practices of living, knowledge, mind wellness and enhanced prana. Yoga stimulates the parasympathetic nervous system (PNS), which help in dissociating one from negative incident and the pains related to it. It educates us that we are even more than the various complications of mind-body.

Pain is unavoidable; pain is facultative. You are blessed, undisturbed by worldly workings. Yoga positions enable you to be conscious of your body, your breath and your feelings. One tries to learn not to recognize feelings of discomfort. No matter how severe the discomfort, or how swift the feelings come on, don't stop to combat them throughout the poses. Disassociate yourself from the pain and feelings as they start rising and wither away or fall.

Note also that pregnant women and individuals with some form of illness must heed recommendations from their physicians before beginning the exercise work. Those with polycystic ovarian syndrome (PCOS), fibroids, or other medical problem may experience severe bleeding if the postures are performed during the menstrual period. Consequently, correct information should be given on how these postures can be proceeded throughout periods.

Spiritual Meanings of Yoga Postures

Yoga is deeply embedded in spiritualism and several of the poses have a lead to greater muscle strength and elongation. Certain poses emphasize energy, such as Warrior, and several emphasize modesty, including such Child. This ancient method using different poses reaches further into the relationship between mind, body, and spirit than the standard gym workout routine.

Almost all the poses performed in yoga stem from Hatha yoga. Such exercises are recognized as "asanas." Many of the best-known asanas performed in yoga have a story behind them. A few obtain their motivation from the animal species, others from the Earth, while others from traditional spiritual stories. Knowing the meaning behind the poses will help connect you with the spiritual dimension of yoga.

Warrior Pose

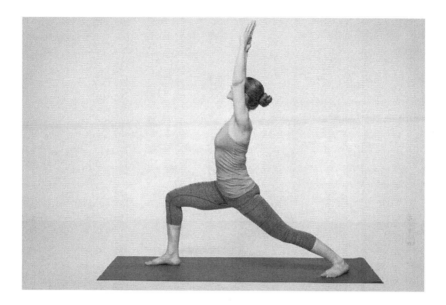

Types of the Warrior pose mostly come from the traditional tale of a warrior named, Virabhadra, the youngest child of the Hindu god, Shiva. Shiva was furious and ripped out a curl of his hair, tossing it to the ground. The hair transformed into an amazingly strong warrior, Virabhadra, who used moral passion to kill his rivals. The poses of the Warrior are physical expressions of this mighty warrior. They are supposed to signify the ego and surmounting hypocrisy.

Tree Pose

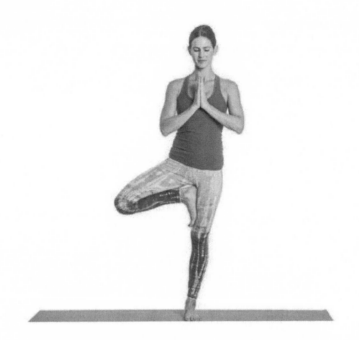

This pose stems from a saga poem by Ramayana. In a portion of the narrative, the devil king, Ravana, catches a lady named, Sita, and keeps her captive in his fortress, attempting to induce her to ignore her banished husband, Rama. Persuaded that Rama will arrive and save her, Sita finds comfort outside the palace among the trees, where she prays and waits patiently for Rama to protect her.

The pose is indicative of Sita's great patience and belief in expecting her banished husband to arrive. At one particular moment, the trees talk to her, saying, "Remain still, little sister. Be relaxed and consistent, like us. Weather changes, we know, we know. This confinement isn't forever. Stay still and memorize Rama." One of the objectives during Tree pose is to remain deeply entrenched in the ground through your foot and retain the pose patiently.

Child's Pose

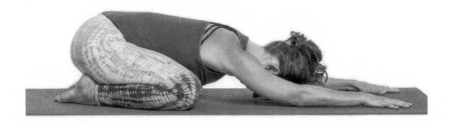

Although this might sound like one of the easiest yoga poses, there's far more than meets the eye. In Child's pose, you lie on the floor with your hands stretched forward and your legs wedged beneath you. This pose symbolizes and brings forth your relation to the childish feeling of capitulation. The overall aim is to be in a form of non-doing, as per Yoga Journal.

This is an essential pose, particularly if you're depressed or strung out. There is a reliance on appropriate breathing that further enhances the relationship between mind and body, helping introduce you to a sense of consciousness to completely loosen up your body.

Corpse Pose

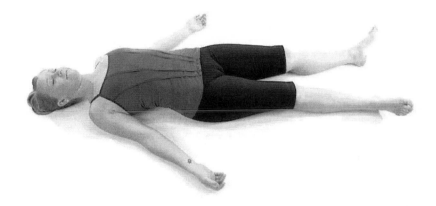

Shava Sana, or Corpse pose, is normally the very last pose in a lesson of yoga. It's a pose for stress relief, done on floor while on your back. It is intended to simulate death. It's essential to keep in mind that the yogic variant of death differs from the Western view. Death is often seen as the maximum degree of life, and why preparation for it is important.

Psychic Development

**"Be thy prophecy master. Learn how to
manage the denser
natural forces and make things,
happenings, living and
working conditions you desire in
your physical existence."**

Psychic Development is the aspect of Yoga that focuses on psychological and psychic capacities. Man is a psychic entity, and thus he psychically (implicitly and explicitly) constructs his world.

The components, items, persons, and situations in human existence are usually drawn into the subconsciousness by mental regularities. Humans tend to attract friends, achievement, and opportunities to themselves or continue to drive them away (unintentionally) because of the psychic law. The rule of mind (since the beginning of the world) is the law of psychic stimulation, and it works exactly like the force of gravitation or electricity. Really! The brain's power is especially potent; it is this that generates the world's physical ailments.

The mind behaves opposite to you or about you; it works for you if you understand how and when to use. It will show you anything you desire, from wellness and riches to sickness and misery. Training in Psychic Development comprises the principles of world materialization and also the training of mantra (scientific sound formulas), pranayama (deep breathing), comprehensive visual analytics, and relaxation techniques that;

- serve to enhance psychological defenses which become less sensitive to adverse vibrations
- tend to help in changing and improve one's living contextual factors by countering and developing mental patterns
- help to bring safety, serenity, and comfort
- are an important instrument in spiritual growth
- offer rarely gained knowledge of the foundation of universe formation
- provide a mantra with defined outcomes and demonstrated sound power on the heart and brain
- provide pranayama (deep breathing) to improve one 's resilience to negative internal and external effects
- involve psychological exercises and guided visual analytics

It is your mental rhythm and emotions that build objects, from which you gain physical ownership in your daily life in the universe. When thought processes became more inventive, their inertial power begins to attract and build, operating on the items, persons and circumstances required for your opinions to eventuate into actual fact.

This energy is well within each one of you, but like everything else in the world, it needs planning and practice in order to allow you to use these forces for productive purposes.

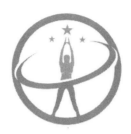

Chapter 5:
Yoga and Pain

Yoga is an extensive system of exercises and a philosophy that comes from India. Hatha Yoga is the most popular and well recognized type of yoga, involving physical postures, different breathing strategies, and relaxation techniques. Yoga is an increasingly common method of exercise and self-care accessed via online yoga classes via gyms, yoga studios, community centers, hospitals, schools and at even home.

Yoga and pain

Yoga has both physical and mental effects and can be effective in pain relief, but yoga is not a quick recovery treatment. Owing to the popular emphasis on air, body, and present moment consciousness, yoga has many of the same benefits as mindfulness practice. Since yoga is also a physical activity, many people consider it more available than the conventional forms of meditation done in silence.

Yoga is especially useful in facilitating relaxation when dealing with tension and agitation. Traditionally, yoga acts as a "warm up: of sorts for the meditation practice of organized sitting and recumbent mindfulness. Yoga can also improve body strength and helps eliminate depression.

Yoga is effective when it comes to managing some of the mechanical factors of pain, for example when tight muscles lead to discomfort. However, practicing yoga improperly or without adequate supervision can also in the short term worsen the discomfort, given that evidence indicates yoga to be as healthy as normal treatment and exercise. Trying to come up with a useful yoga routine takes greater care and expertise when you have a chronic pain condition, particularly when your nervous system is hypersensitive and you are prone to flare-ups.

It is necessary to start gradually with yoga, and to be successful, it must be practiced frequently and with awareness.

What is the evidence for yoga's effectiveness when you have pain?

Yoga improves the pain impairment and mood of those with chronic pain. It's impact can be called "moderate", approximately equivalent to Cognitive Behavior Therapy (CBT). Yoga is one of the treatments the American Pain Society recommends for people with low back pain who do not benefit from certain self-care methods.

Most research is on the effects of yoga in people with chronic back pain, while bowel irritable syndrome, arthritis, headache / migraine, carpal tunnel syndrome and fibromyalgia can also be helped. We do need more high-quality research to establish which pain conditions yoga is most beneficial for, as well as which forms of yoga are best suited for pain. So far, Iyengar Yoga, Hatha Yoga and Viniyoga have the most scientific evidence, but we really do not completely understand how yoga benefits such people.

Emerging research indicates that beyond pain relief, yoga could help us manage more effectively how we think and behave, both mentally and physically. It may improve muscle strength, reduce inflammation, encourage relaxation, foster self-control, increase the release of pain-relieving endorphins, and boost self-confidence.

How to choose a Yoga teacher and class?

Yoga is an unregulated industry at present. Unlike health professions like nursing, physiotherapy or psychology, anyone can call themselves an instructor of yoga. Some professional yoga instructors may recommend a class for you and some offer Yoga Therapy or Restorative Yoga courses especially for those with disabilities, chronic pain, or chronic disease. By seeking a yoga instructor who has trained to become a yoga therapist and is registered with either the (IAYT) - the acronym of International Association of Yoga Therapists - or the (AAYT) - the acronym of Australasian Association of Yoga Therapists, you may get the best advice for your pain condition.

Can anyone do yoga?

Yes, yoga is good for all, but you need to talk to the instructor before starting. There are several different yoga types and at this point in your life not all lessons will be right for you. Start with a private class if you have unique needs, preferably with a Yoga Therapist.

Can I do yoga at home?

It is not recommended to begin yoga practice at home without a yoga teacher's supervision. If you find it challenging to get to a class, you can opt to do it in the comfort of your home. Many yoga instructors are willing to conduct a private practice, if you are approved be to access the poses. If you have more yoga experience, your instructor give recommendations as to what activities are acceptable for you at home.

Do I need to tell my health care professional I am doing yoga?

Yes! Before you begin yoga classes, it is important to advise your health care professional. You want to ask your health care provider to share the details of your condition with your yoga teacher / therapist.

All about pain

For centuries, scientists and physicians have believed that pain is related to the body's structure. In bulging spinal discs, muscle strain, and diseases they have searched for the cause of chronic pain. Nonetheless, more recent work points to another cause of chronic pain: the specific biology of feelings, emotions, perceptions, and memories. Most chronic pain has its origin in a physical accident or disease, but it is caused by how the initial trauma not only affects the body but also the nature of the bond between the mind and the body.

The nature of chronic pain is good news indeed. It means that the only chance to heal the body is with surgery, pain medicine or physical therapy. First recognizing chronic pain as an experience of the mind-body and then using the healing practices toolbox of yoga — including relaxation techniques and restorative poses — you will find true relief from pain and start reclaiming your life.

THE PROTECTIVE PAIN RESPONSE

Your ability to reduce and control pain is be crucial to recognizing the difference between acute and chronic pain. Let us start by reviewing the basic pain responses: feeling, stress and suffering.

The defensive response to pain starts when the body faces some physical danger, such as cutting, burning, or an inflamed muscle. Specialized nerves sense this threat and transmit it through the spinal cord up to the brain, where the danger signals are converted into perceptions of pain, among others. The brain's emotion-processing fields often get the message, causing a wide range of responses, from fear to anger. Your thoughts and feelings about the physical experiences of pain, combined, make up the suffering dimension of the full perception of pain.

The threat signals are simultaneously directed to certain areas of the brain to help the body initiate an emergency stress response, by coordinating the activities of the nervous system, endocrine system, and immune system to help you act. The reaction to emergency stress causes a cascade of physiological changes that will give you the strength and concentration to defend yourself against a life-threatening risk.

Even after the danger is gone, the reaction to the pain is not over. The mind and body are keen to make sure that in the future you know how to defend yourself from this danger. The nervous system then begins learning from this experience. Any form of injury or disease will affect the way the nervous system experiences pain, including one that is short-lived or appears to be completely healed.

UNDERSTANDING CHRONIC PAIN

Chronic pain varies in three essential ways from acute pain. First, the body becomes more sensitive to danger, transmitting signals of danger to the brain even when there is a slight or non-existent threat. Second, the brain becomes more likely to perceive a circumstance as dangerous, and feelings as painful, resulting in pain reactions out of proportion to any actual danger. Finally, the distinctions between the many aspects of the pain response — feeling, suffering, and stress — get distorted with repeated pain experiences. The mind and body have learned all too well in most cases of chronic pain how to sense the slightest sign of a threat and stage a complete defensive response in all of its glory.

So, the things that make medicine so effective in helping us endure acute situations and treat short-term pain are the same things that make chronic pain so difficult and lasting. The pain you feel can represent a hostile response of the mind-body which has become over-protective.

PAIN AGAIN

Why does past suffering making you more prone to future pain? You can thank one of our nervous system's great wonders: the capacity to learn as a response to experiences. The ability is called neuroplasticity. The nervous system gets better at detecting danger and generating the defensive pain response through repeated experiences of pain. And, sadly, in the case of chronic pain, paradoxically learning from practice and becoming "better" at pain means more pain, not less.

This concept is shared by both of yoga and modern science: current pain and suffering have its origins in past pain, trauma, loss, stress, and illness. Medical science explains the learning process from previous experience using terminology like neuroplasticity; yoga invented the phrase samskara. Samskaras are the experiences of the body and mind that shape the way we perceive the moment. Samskaras keep you trapped, feel the same feelings, think the same thoughts, and even feel the same pain.

Not only do Samskaras lead to suffering, but they also lead to great change. Good interactions do just as trauma, pain, sickness, and stress leave marks on the body and mind. You become what you are practicing. Training is a lifelong process and none of the improvements you have made will be lasting. It is possible to harness neuroplasticity for treatment. Your body and mind have known how to "do" chronic pain, and there is little new to teach it.

UNLEARNING PAIN THROUGH RELAXATION

By helping you to turn chronic pain-and-stress responses into mind and body responses to "chronic healing," yoga helps to reduce chronic pain suffering. Your body and mind have built-in healing responses that are as strong as their protective reactions to pain and stress. Whether it's a gratitude meditation, a calming posture that helps your body and mind feel at ease, or a breathing exercise that enhances the body's flow of energy — they all have the purpose of taking you back home to your normal sense of well-being.

Specifically, relaxation has been shown to be a remedy for chronic pain. It switches off the stress response and directs the energy of the body to the processes of development, repair, digestion, immune function, and self-nurturing. The calming response unravels the samskaras of the mind-body that contribute to pain and provide the basis for healing habits. The mind and body may go to rest in a sense of comfort rather than chronic emergency when we regular practice relaxation. Here we will look at a method of breathing and some poses of restorative yoga that facilitate the response to relaxation.

BREATHING THE WHOLE BODY

Breathing the body is a meditation technique derived from the conventional technique of yoga nidra (yogic sleep) and the body-scan technique taught for people with chronic pain by Jon Kabat-Zinn's mindfulness-based stress reduction programs. Begin any comfortable pose like Savasana (Corpse pose) for relaxation. Put your hands on your chest and feel the air circulation. Note the rising and dropping of the belly, and consider the air moving inside and outside the body. Direct your breath right at feelings of discomfort. Assume the breath is softening the stress and pain.

Imagine inhaling and exhaling from various parts of your body — as if your nostrils were moving to that part. Start with the feet. Assume that the breath coming through your body goes through the soles and is leaving your body through your heels. Note any feelings there. Feel the surge of energy in your feet as you imagine. Now for other areas of the body, repeat this visualization: the lower legs, elbows, and upper legs. Then your middle back, lower back, upper back and knees. Next your stomach and your chest. Don't neglect your upper arms, your elbows, your lower arms, your legs, your neck. What about the back, face, and crown of the head.

Do not miss a place that feels stressed, awkward, or painful. There are some things you can do to feel more at ease. Next, stay with the visualization and the sensations of discomfort or pain and direct the breath. Imagine the air dissolving stress and pain or massaging it. Imagine the stress or discomfort softening. Find the gap of pain within. Next, between the unpleasant area and a more relaxed area, shift your mind back and forth. Breathe in the unpleasant area a few times, then breathe out into another area for the next few breaths. Going back and forth like this will instruct the mind how to pay less attention to sensations of pain. You can practice a healthy sort of distraction by consciously changing your attention while still present in your body.

Once you have worked your way through the entire body, allow yourself to feel the oxygen coming in through your mouth, nose, and throat. Imagine the breathing sensation across the whole body, as though the body were expanding softly as you inhale and contracting as you exhale. Experience the flow of energy through the whole body or imagine it.

A RESTORATIVE YOGA ROUTINE FOR CHRONIC PAIN

The soothing relaxation response is converted to restorative yoga by integrating gentle yoga poses with mindful breathing. Below you'll learn four poses of restorative yoga that can be done either alone or in a series.

Many factors make restorative yoga so calming. Each pose is intended to last longer than a few breaths. You can remain for 10 minutes or even longer in a restore pose. The stillness allows even the deepest layers of tension to fall away from the body. Use props for restorative poses to support your body, including a chair, wall, pillows, sofa, towels, blankets, or bolsters specifically made for restorative yoga. They help make it feel effortless, so your body can let go indefinitely.

In more active yoga, the way you pose should not incur strong sensations of strength or elongation. Stretching and strengthening are both sources of stress on the body, although healthy. They are really a nice kind of stress, challenging the body to adapt to a pose's challenges. Restorative yoga is all about taking away stress and tension.

Though these poses may look like you are not doing much, it is far from the reality. The body rests on restorative yoga but it activates the mind. A pose's breathing elements make restorative yoga an active method of concentrating the mind on calming thoughts, feelings, and emotions.

The order of the poses described here is one possible sequence. When you master the poses, you may find that your body prefers a particular set, or you would rather remain in one pose for longer than perform multiple poses for shorter periods of time. Restorative poses can also be incorporated into an active yoga session.

NESTING POSE

Nesting pose provides a feeling of safety and nourishment. This can also be a position in which you sleep comfortably, making it an ideal pose to learn if you have insomnia or other sleeping difficulties.

Lie on your side with your legs bent and pulled in towards your stomach. Lay your head on a mattress and put a pillow or bolster between your knees. Rest your arms in any place they feel most relaxed. If available, you might place another bolster or pillow behind your back for an additional sense of comfort.

Rest at your breath's normal rhythm, tracking every inhalation and exhalation as it passes through your body. Take comfort from this action in its simplicity and effortlessness.

SUPPORTED BOUND ANGLE POSE

This posture relieves tension in the belly, chest, and shoulders that can otherwise hinder breathing. Lean a bolster over a block (or other help such as books or the phone. Sit in diamond shape with your legs in front of the bolster. Place a pillow or roller under each knee and outer thigh, knowing that the legs are fully supported in the knees, thighs or hips without heavy stretching or strain. Bend down onto the bolster, protecting your lower back to the back of the skull. Rest your arms wherever you feel most relaxed.

Note now the front of your entire body relaxes and expands as you slowly inhale. Follow the feeling and experience the breathable comfort in the front of the body.

SUPPORTED BACKBEND POSE

A supported backbend is the opening pose of the heart that strengthens your ability to accept life and not allow obstacles to detach you from life — including pain. This position often helps alleviate chronic back pain and shoulders tension easily, trying to undo postural habits arising from spending a lot of time on a desk, phone, or driving.

Place a bolster, a collection of pillows, or sheets below bent knees while sitting. A rolled pillow, towel or blanket can be placed behind; when you lie back, the upper rib cage will be covered, not only the lower back. If you need additional assistance underneath the lower back and lower rib cage, roll a small towel to help the natural spine curve. To support your head and back, place a folded towel or simple blanket at whatever height is most comfortable.

This pose increases breath flow in the upper chest, rib cage, and abdomen. Let yourself experience this movement as you inhale and exhale. Imagine getting the heart center breathing in and out. Try to imagine the air moving in your heart and to the lungs while you breathe, then through the middle of your heart as you exhale back out of the lungs.

SUPPORT FOR FORWARD BEND

This type of pose relaxes the back and hip, unraveling the tension on the spine from the everyday activities. Hugging a bolster and leaning your head on it imparts a natural sense of comfort and security.

Sit on the floor, cross-legged. Lean forward onto a couch, chair, or stack of pillows, blankets, or cushions to assist. Place one end on the couch and the other on the lap, chair, or stack holder, if you have a bolster. Whatever help you can get, lay your head on it. If you are using a bolster, you can hug it in some way that feels normal, turning your head toward the side. Make sure the support you use is high and strong enough to sustain you, without causing back or hip strain. You will need more help if you encounter a heavy stretch that is difficult to bear.

When doing these types of poses, with every breath, the abdomen, back and throat will expand and contract. As you inhale and exhale, note the motion of the whole body. Softly pressing your belly and chest into the bolster or pillow as you inhale. Let your breath intensify your feeling of being hugged.

Relaxation from these poses will help you on the road to ending your suffering. Yoga will show you how to concentrate your mind so you can improve your physical pain. It can give you back the sense of confidence, power, and strength you need to move beyond your chronic pain experience.

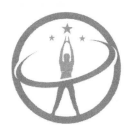

Chapter 6:
Beginners Exercises to Heal Back-Pain Scoliosis at Home

Scoliosis develops a lateral curvature of the spine, resulting in irritation, fatigue, and a shift in the way a person moves. Workout and meditation are important aspects of rehabilitation. Scoliosis can be in moderate conditions with different movements and stretching alone, thereby removing any need for surgeries.

Among the medical factors that promote scoliosis, teenage idiopathic scoliosis is perhaps the most common type. This type grows as the adult continues to expand. It and influences 2-3 percent of the population. Although researchers have found proof to support particular scoliosis movements, it is a great idea to talk to a doctor or physiotherapist about the right stretches and activities for an individual with scoliosis.

Stretches and exercises for scoliosis

The proper workouts for scoliosis rely on where the scoliosis curve is located. Individuals with lumbar scoliosis must concentrate on lower back workouts, while individuals with thoracic scoliosis must work out the shoulders.

For individuals with scoliosis, physicians can prescribe the following specific exercises and stretches:

1: Pelvic tilts

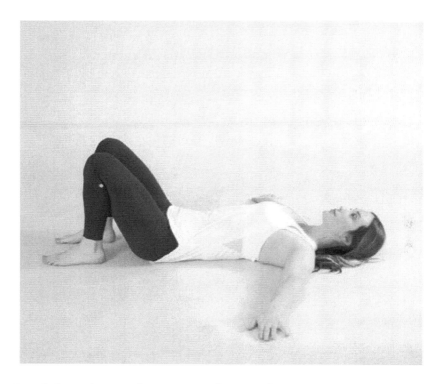

A pelvic twist tends to extend tense hip muscle groups and lower back muscles.

- Lay flat on the ground with your palms on your back and knees bent.
- Tighten your stomach muscles while flattening your back toward the floor.
- Maintain for 5 seconds with regular breathing.
- Release.
- Perform two sets of 10.

2: *Arm and leg raises*

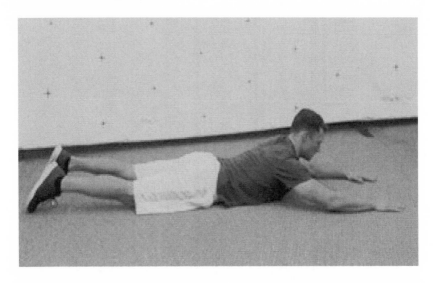

Individual can flatten their lower back with leg and arm raises. To perform the raises:

- Lie on the front with your forehead on the floor.
- Extend your arms above your head, placing the hands flat on the floor. Keep your legs tight.
- Pick one arm off the floor.
- Hold for one or two full breaths, then drop the arm down.
- Repeat it with each leg and arm.
- Do a set of 15 per leg.

3: Cat-Camel

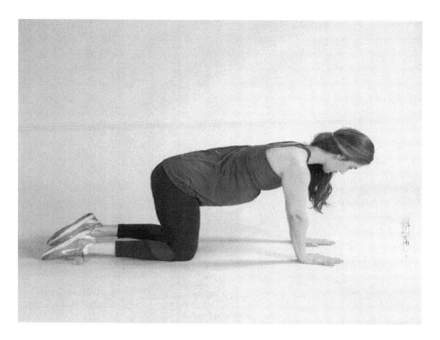

The Cat-Camel can assist to maintain a stable and trauma-free spine. To make pose:

- Start on your hands and knees, making sure that your back is flat and your head and neck are relaxed.
- Breathe slowly and then pull the stomach muscles in and up, while bending the spine.
- Exhale the stomach muscles and loosen them, lower the buttocks, let the abdomen fall and raise the head to upward.
- Perform two sets of 10.

4: *Bird-Dog*

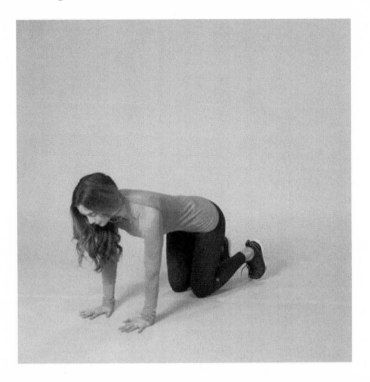

The Bird-Dog is yet another yoga pose. For the workout:

- Start with your back flat and on the hands and knees.
- Put your hands beneath your shoulders, with the knees immediately below your hips.
- Extend one arm straight out and forward while pulling straight to the opposite side.
- Breathe normally and hold for 5 seconds.
- Move the opposite arm and leg.
- Conduct repetitions of 10–15 per side.

5: *Latissimus dorsi stretch*

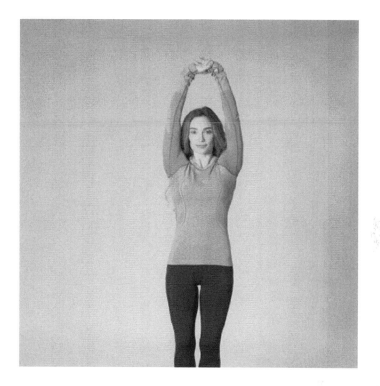

Through this pose, you will stretch the latissimus dorsi — the biggest muscle in the upper body. Thoracic scoliosis influences certain muscles specifically. Lumbar scoliosis may cause extreme tension which extends to the latissimus dorsi.

To do a latissimus dorsi stretch:

- Stand in a neutral position, with a proper stance.
- Hold the feet shoulder-width apart and bend the knees moderately.
- After putting both hands above your head, grasp your right arm with your left hand.

- Bend marginally to the right leg, until you notice a strain along the body's left hand.
- Hold for one or two minutes, then return to the initial position with on left foot.
- Switch to the other side.
- Perform 5–10 repetitions on each side.

6: Abdominal press

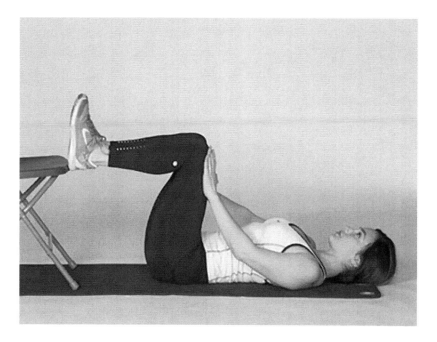

Having strong abdominal muscles can assist in taking pressure off the back-muscle pressure. It can assist a person in maintain good posture too.

To do an abdominal press:

- With a flat back on the ground, draw your feet up with legs bent.
- Hold the back in a position that is stable, stress free.
- Raise the lower legs off the floor until you reach an angle of 90 degrees.
- Using the hands to press back on the knees while at the same time raising the legs towards the hands to

stimulate the abdominal muscles. This is a stable workout, and while you are pushing, the legs and arms do not move.

- Take 3 full breaths and then relax.
- Perform two sets of 10.

7: *Practicing good posture*

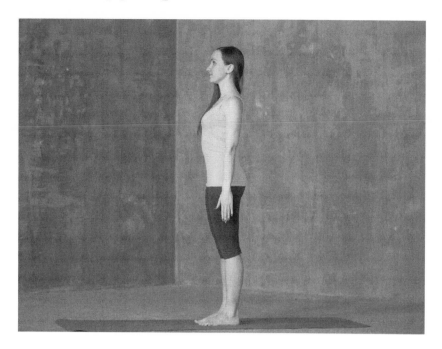

Healthy posture can reduce muscle stress and pain. An individual should reconfigure his or her body many times a day to assist them in learning to stand spontaneously with proper posture.

To have a good posture when standing:

- Drop the shoulders down and back
- Position your ears over your shoulders
- Pull the chin in gently so it does not move forward or too far down
- Slightly lower your stomach
- Unlock the knees a bit

Hold the back flat, with the ears over the shoulders while seated. The legs will be straight, not crossed. This will assist in checking the body for signs of distress. For example, some people tense their shoulders unintentionally or lean marginally to one side, particularly when they are in pain or under strain.

Targeted exercise programs

Doctors and researchers have developed several targeted scoliosis programs. For example, the **Scientific Exercises Approach to Scoliosis (SEAS)** is an individualized program that teaches a person to steadily correct movement issues and change the position of their spine.

The most effective fitness regimen depends on the form and severity of scoliosis. If a doctor suggests a particular fitness routine, inquire what home workouts are appropriate to perform, and what activities to stop.

Exercises to avoid

Some practices and treatments may make the effects of scoliosis worse or raise the risk of secondary injury. Scoliosis sufferers should prevent:

- Holding the neck angled slightly, as when using a smartphone, and when the head faces downwards.

- Soccer and other high-contact games are unsafe for individuals with scoliosis.
- Ballet and gymnastics will harm the thoracic spine as well.
- Extending the torso repeatedly is not wise, as in some yoga poses, ballet moves, and gymnastics moves.
- Exposing the body to repetitive leaping or moving impacts is undesirable. The usual culprits involve trampolines, riding horseback and walking long distances on rough surfaces.

Other Tips

In addition to exercise, a range of home management solutions may help.

Bracing can prevent a deterioration of the spinal curve, decrease pain and enhance mobility. The best bracing technique depends on a person's form of scoliosis so speak to a doctor before you use a brace.

Choosing the right furniture: an ergonomic chair or mattress will help to balance the back and spine, thereby lowering discomfort.

Massage: Some people find that massage helps relieve discomfort from scoliosis.

Summary

The spectrum ranges from moderate to severe scoliosis. Observation and home workouts are enough, in some cases, to remedy a spinal curve. In more serious cases, a patient may require more care, including bracing, surgery, and physical therapy. Since types scoliosis can impair the stability and general well-being of a person, so it is important to see a specialist on scoliosis before choosing a course of action.

9 Yoga Poses for Upper Back Pain

The stress of sitting at a desk or peering down at your mobile phone can result in severe back pain, especially in the upper part. To get rid of the pain or anxiety, perform yoga poses.

The upper back is susceptible to becoming tightened. Our thoracic spine is the middle portion connected to the ribs, which inherently renders this part of the spine less flexible than the cervical spine above and the lumbar spine beneath. Continuous sitting and staring at operating systems negatively affects posture, resulting in shoulder, chest, and neck stiffness.

Nine yoga poses will enable us to counteract the symptoms of sitting and improper positions by relaxing the tense chest muscles, shoulders and upper back muscles around the thoracic spine. A yoga mat and two yoga blocks are all you require.

Cat-Cow | 8 breaths

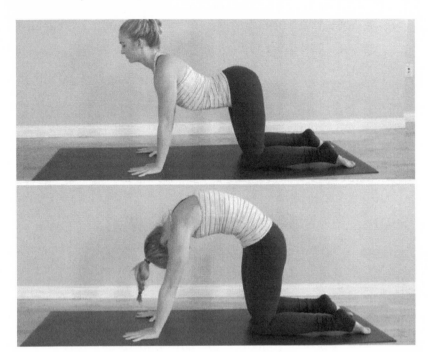

These paired yoga poses help in warming the whole body, while at the same time relaxing the rhomboids and trapezoids, easing stiffness in the upper back.

- Start with your hands and legs in a tabletop posture. Move your shoulders across your wrists and your thighs over your knees.

- Flip your tailbone towards the heavens on an inhalation, trying to lower your abdomen to the ground to enter the pose of the cow. Keep squeezing closed your hands and hold your neck down. Feel an extension throughout the abdomen.

- Breathe out deeply towards the sky and then round your spinal column to get into cat pose. Direct your navel up and down to your spinal column as you twist your jawline to your chest and look at your abdomen. Push the floor and perceive an extension in the middle and upper back.
- Perform eight breath sessions in your cow and cat poses.

Thread the Needle | 8 breaths per side

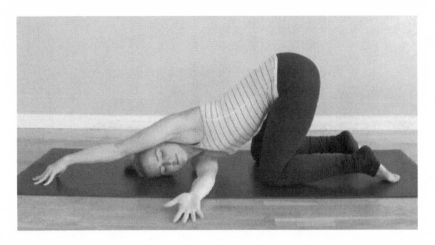

This pose releases rhomboid, trapezoid and shoulders friction.

- Begin in a tabletop pose, folding your wrists underneath your shoulders.
- Breathe in as you raise your right hand from the mat and bend it toward heaven.
- Breathe out and put your right hand under your left arm. Put your right shoulder at the temple on the mat to relax.
- Move your left fingers up your mat and feel a pull through your right shoulder blade.
- Keep at it for eight deep breaths, then return to tabletop and switch sides.

Double V Pose | 8 breaths per side

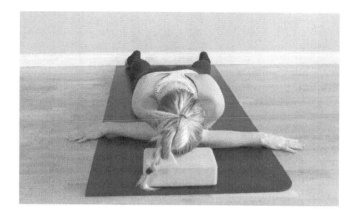

This position alleviates stress in the shoulders, rhomboids, trapezius, latissimus dorsi, and also the neck.

- Put a bock on upper edge of the mat and keep lying on your abdomen.
- Prop yourself up on the forearms and continue to work your biceps.
- Flip your right forearm over your mat, as your fingertips move to the mat's opposite side.
- Flip your left forearm towards the front of the right forearm and place your left fingertips to the right side of the mat. Move your chest until your forearms are right over them.
- Move your fingertips to the sides of your mat, so you can cross your arms beneath your chest.
- Take your forehead to the block to relax and shut your eyes. Keep on for eight minutes, then change sides.

Child's Pose with Side Stretch | 8 breaths per side

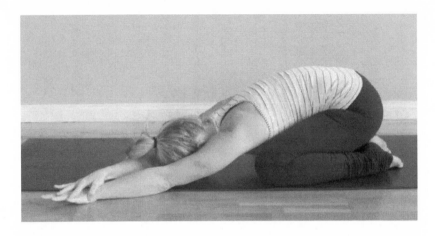

This pose extends the muscles behind the ribs, helping to relieve stress in the lats.

- Begin with a tabletop pose, on your arms and knees.
- Put your feet next to each other and your knees far to your mat's edges.
- Place your thighs on your heels and then move your arms to the upper edge of the mat and bend your chest along the ground. Let the forehead rest on the mat.
- Move your palms down to the right side of the mat and push your hips softly to the left for a stretch across your left leg.
- Keep on for eight breaths, then switch hands.

Eagle Arms | 8 breaths

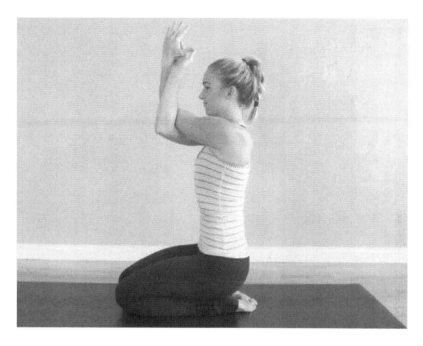

This binding pose alleviates stress in the space between the rhomboids, traps, and deltoids.

- Sit on a mat with resting arms.
- Tuck your right arm beneath your left one, and then tuck your forearms so they are touched by your palms. If this is not feasible, put each hand on the opposite shoulder.
- Raise the elbows up to the shoulders and push the forearms forward. You should experience a pull across the back and shoulders.
- Hold for eight breaths.

Puppy Pose | 8 breaths

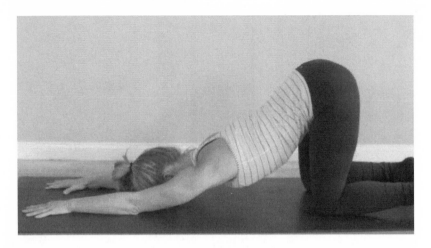

This pose eases stiffness in the trapezius, lats, anterior serratus, chest, and forearms.

- Begin in tabletop pose, with your hips over your knees.
- With your thighs taut, move your arms to the top of your mat and drop your chest to the ground direction. Place your forehead onto the mat to relax.
- Sense a stretching across the lats, arms and shoulders. Hold for eight breaths.

Rabbit Pose | 8 breaths

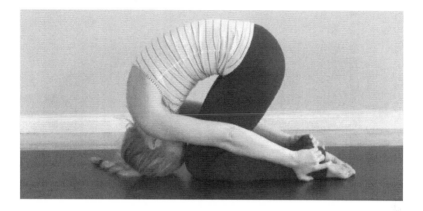

This pose soothes pressure over the shoulders and back.

- Begin to tabletop pose on your hands and knees.
- Pull your legs together the whole time while leaning back on your feet. Then extend your arms to the upper edge of the mat and drop your shoulders to your hips in to reach the posture of the fetus.
- Return your arms to your toes and turn your palms slowing until they are holding your heels. Turn your jaw towards your chest and place the crown of the head on your mat to relax slowly and carefully.
- Holding your feet, breathe in and raise your thighs high into the sky. Please ensure your chin is safely tucked in and prevent any burden on your head. You will sense a stretching all over the spine.
- Retain for eight breaths, then release it and return slowly to the pose of the fetus.

Supine Twist | 8 breaths per side

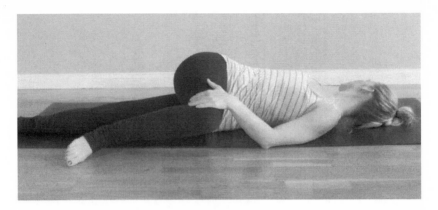

This pose alleviates stress in the chest and arms, and along the backbone.

- lying on the back. cuddle your right knee into the chest.
- With your palm pointing down, meet your right arm out towards the edge of the mat.
- Use your left hand to direct your right leg into a supine bend of your body. Please ensure that your right shoulder rests on the floor. Look right or straight up.
- Continue for eight breaths, then switch hands.

Supported Fish Pose | Relax 2-5 minutes

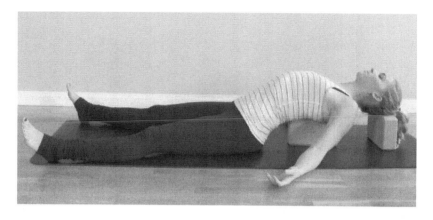

This restorative yoga pose is wonderful to open the chest and shoulders to reduce the severe effects of traveling or staring at your mobile device.

- Place a yoga block at the upper edge of your mat at a minimum or moderate height. Then put another block at the same below vertically under the upper back between the shoulder blades. The blocks must be separated by at least a few inches.
- Arms extend to the side. The head is protected by the upper block.
- Raise your hands with relaxed palms facing up together with your body. Extend your legs. Close your eyes and loosen up for two to five breaths.

8 stretches for the middle back

Discomfort or tightness in the mid back can have a considerable impact on one's lives. Several stretching's can alleviate injuries and discomfort with inflexibility. Back pain, notably short-term pain, is one of world's standard health complaints. A range of factors relate to diet, health problems and incidents.

Symptoms of mid back pain can include:

- Fast, tight pains
- Dull, persistent aches
- Muscle tension or rigidity
- Limited joint mobility

The eight essential exercises are simple to do at home or the office. They can help alleviate mid back pain, relax tight muscles and enhance mobility.

1. Seated twist

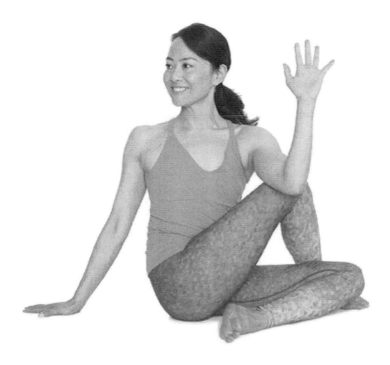

The seated twist extension can assist in determining how stiff the muscles of the mid back are, even while slowly boosting their strength and flexibility in both dimensions.

Poses involving sitting with rounded shoulders can trigger a tightening of the mid-back muscles, restricting the ability of the spinal column to bend. During the pose, you must concentrate on sitting upright, with the back straight and the head neutral.

To perform the seated twist:

- Sit on a bench or chair, with the legs outstretched in front or pointed forward. Pull the shoulder blades together and down while sitting straight.
- Bend slowly toward the left. Put the right hand just outside the left knee and the left hand well behind the back for assistance.
- Keep the pose approximately for twenty or thirty seconds, then switch and repeat the action.
- Perform the stretch on each side four or five times.
- Doing it at a desk can reduce friction in the back that could last all day.

2. Child's Pose

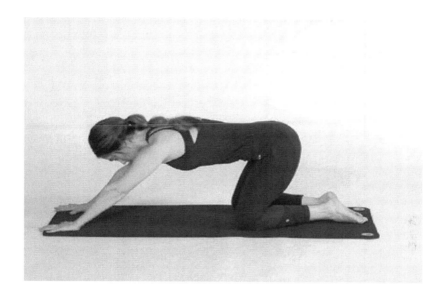

Child's pose is a really easy and calming yoga position. It enables the spine to consciously lengthen while the person is resting over the knees. It will extend the abdominal core muscles connecting the lower back to the long leg bone. Stretching the hands softly over the head extends the latissimus dorsi, the big flat muscle linking the spine with the arms.

To perform the Child's Pose:

Begin in a kneeling posture with the thighs and buttocks resting on the bent legs and feet below.

- Move the knees apart to a convenient point. Then roll the body using on elbows, while pulling back the chest.

- Position the forehead on the ground as comfortable, with the hands extended out in front. The arms must relax while the hands are taut.
- Relax for approximately twenty to thirty seconds.
- Use the hands to help get back upright.

3. Thread the Needle

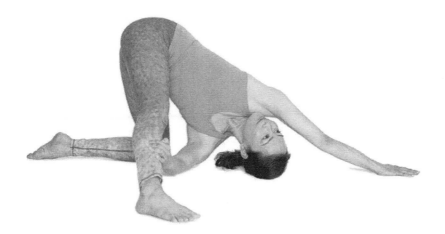

Thread the Needle is a yoga posture that spans the sides of the body to the latissimus dorsi. This extension should assist in releasing the upper back muscles, too. Concentrate on the arms stretched outward and sustaining a relaxed and not uncomfortable position to get maximum benefit.

To perform Thread, the Needle:

- Begin on the arms and knees, with the knees aligned with the thighs just behind the hips and toes.
- Hold the thighs, knees, and feet steady, move the arms out to the front. Maintain your hands taut so you will feel a slight stretching down the sides.
- Push the right arm and move the left arm while twisting the chest. The right hand will lie palm up.

- Keep the right shoulder as low as possible while gently placing the right side of the head on the ground. Look up.
- Maintain the pose for approximately twenty to thirty seconds.
- Move the right arm upwards and gently to the initial spot. Repeat the stretching with left arm.

4. Cat-Cow Pose

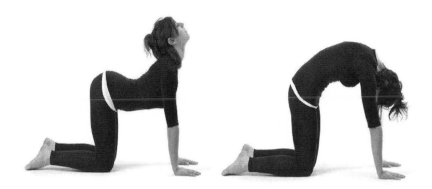

The Cat-Cow pose, like as the Child's pose, is another easy and effective yoga activity. It assists the shoulders and the musculature that runs through the middle of the spine to relieve exertion. Implementing it on a regular basis will progressively increase flexibility.

To perform the Cat-Cow Pose:

- Begin with the knees underneath the thighs and the wrists under the shoulders. Stretch the fingertips and push them with uniform pressure. The backbone will be neutral.

- Inhale and let belly sink toward the floor, while holding out the buttocks. Raise the head and neck, stick out the chest and look straight forward. This is the Cow position.

- Now to another pose. Curve the back like a cat. Flip the pelvis toward the ribs, pushing the blades of the shoulder apart and the abdomen away from the floor. Let head sink to the floor.
- Move five to ten times in these 2 positions.

5. *Latissimus dorsi stretch*

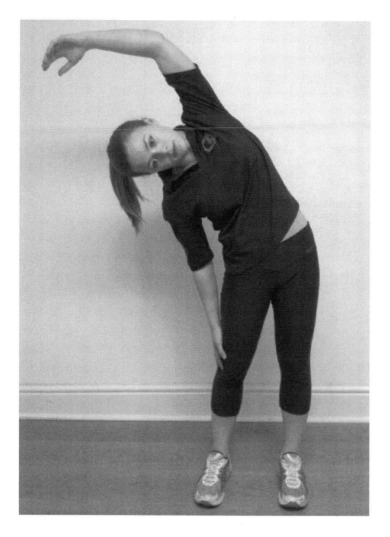

You can do this while sitting or standing. Maintaining the backbone stretched and the chest elevated is significant. This simple activity also extends the muscles in the serratus underneath the hands.

To perform the latissimus dorsi stretch:

- Standing up or sitting down, lift your right hand straight over your head.
- Flex the elbow, as the right arm falls to the upper back.
- Position the left arm onto the right elbow and pull the right arm softly to the left.
- Flex the body in a lean line to the left even when pulling the right elbow, ensuring that it is not leaning forward or backward.
- Continue the workout approximately twenty to thirty seconds, then return back to the other position.

6. Passive backbend

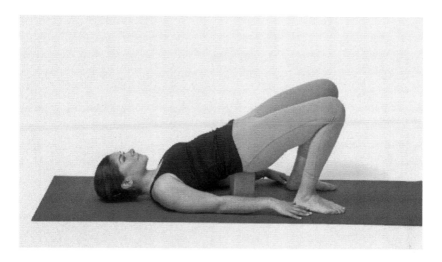

This simplistic pose can give considerable comfort. It expands the muscle groups of the scalene neck, the serratus. and the chest. The submissive backbend includes putting a supportive surface, including a block, a foam roller or a tightly rolled towel or mat under the back.

To perform the exercise:

- Put the block on the ground under the buttocks and retain the pose.
- If it requires an uncomfortable extension, put something below the head.
- Take the arms off the chest and lie at such an inclination of 45 degrees.
- Maintain the stance for approximately one to two minutes.

7. *Cobra Pose*

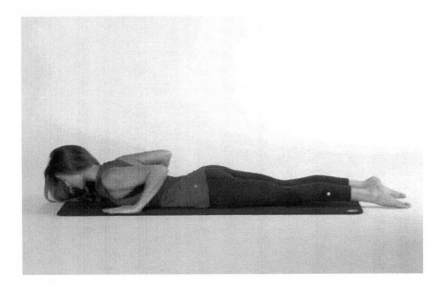

The priority of this yoga pose is on effective back bending. Individuals with middle back pain likely won't go very far. Don't extend beyond what is comfortable.   Back bending assists in stretching the chest while reinforcing muscle groups in the spinal column.

To perform the Cobra Pose:

- Lying face down on the ground stretch the legs, with the tops of the feet relaxed.
- Place your hands beneath your shoulders, with your fingers forward. Flex the elbows and maintain your hands into the body.
- Start engaging the muscles in the buttocks and legs to assist in pushing the legs and feet into the ground. This

is crucial because it assists the lower back while extending the spinal column and lifting the chest.

- Use the hands to raise the head slowly, then the chest off the ground.

- Flex the back as feasible by flattening the hands and pulling the chest further from the ground. Some individuals cannot do this — just go as far as you can.

- Maintain the pose for approximately twenty to thirty seconds. Return to normal, complete the stretching in 2 or 4 stages.

8. Bridge

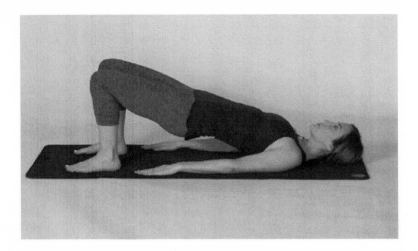

The bridge can reinforce the muscle groups running all along spinal column and also those in the buttocks and abdomen. Implementing this extension routinely, while sitting in a chair or standing up, could even assist an individual in retain a strong upright position.

To perform the bridge:

- Sit with the legs bent. The feet must rest on the ground, pulled in as near to the buttocks as feasible, with the hands to the sides.
- Trying to squeeze the buttocks, elevate the pelvis towards the ceiling and lift the torso till the back is off the ground. The shoulders now hold the weight of the body.
- Hold that pose for five seconds, focusing on pressing the buttocks.

- Bend the torso slowly, allowing each vertebra to touch the ground until the back returns to a flat position.
- Repeat twelve to fifteen times per series, and perform up to three sets progressively.

Tips for managing back pain

Easy measures may help alleviate discomfort and lessen or prevent recurrence:

Stay mobile. Movement ease rigidity. Seek to remain healthy, and then do some gentle flexing and some type of work as possible.

Medication. Over-the-counter pain medicine including ibuprofen or acetaminophen can assist in alleviating discomfort quickly and lessen inflammation.

Complementary therapies. A few people find that massage, herbal remedies, or transcutaneous stimuli of electrical nerves (TENS) support back pain for a lengthy period.

Posture. Learn a healthy seated pose. Seek not to slouch and take daily rests. Make sure chairs and work areas are comfortable and set up properly. Some find adequate support from standing desks.

Yoga and Pilates. Most individuals find that practices like yoga and Pilates significantly improve posture and alleviate backache.

5 Yoga Poses to Ease Lower Back Pain

The lower back or lumbar zone seems to be vulnerable at any stage of life. Either were going to have to sit up quite a lot during the day or carry a lot, and the lumbar zone may get directly impacted. In either case, lower back pain can have severe implications for your frame of mind and your day. Yoga provides a good cure for discomfort and is an excellent preventive treatment.

There are 5 positions of yoga that serve to alleviate lower back pain and assist in reducing mild headaches.

1. Supine Twist

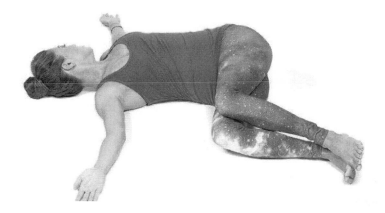

Twisting the spinal column affects the entire back and also the neck, as a wonderful stress reliever. You lie down, rest and then let gravity support you.

- Lie on your back, put your hands on the ground in a T-shape and bring your knees to your chest. Bend both knees to the left and maintain the neck position. The eyes are looking away from the knees.
- Hold your shoulders on the ground and if the top of the knees raise up too far, you can put brace between them.
- Retain the pose between one to four minutes and perform the exercise on the other side.

2. *Sphinx Pose*

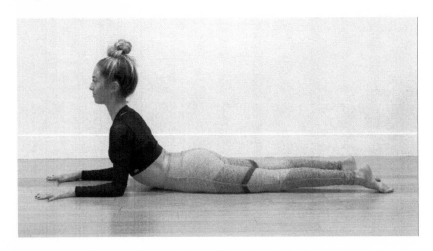

The Sphinx is a wonderful posture as a tonic for the spinal column and to stimulate the sacral-lumbar arch. The lower back straightens when we are seated a lot, causing discomfort. The Sphinx pose favors the natural lower back circumference.

- Begin by lying on the abdomen, separating your feet thigh-width, with the elbows below your shoulders. If your lower back gets stressed, put your elbows ahead a bit.

- Put a block underneath the elbows if you seek a broader bend. Remain in the position for one to three minutes and come out by bending your upper body to the ground. Stay as you require and then perform the Child's pose for short breaths.

3. Thread the Needle Pose

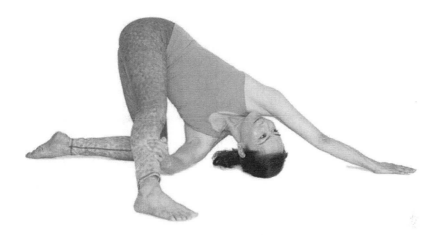

If the thighs are stiff, the activity occurs from the back, resulting in back pain. This can assist in alleviating lower back pain when the thighs and leg muscles are responsive, as the body has a good range of motion. This position extends the thighs, the lower back, and the backbone. Pigeon pose is also a mild, refined version.

- To get started, lie flat and with the soles of the feet on the ground, thigh-distance apart. Position your right ankle on the left thigh, keeping your foot stretched across the position. Place your right arm between the knees and your left arm above the left calf.

- Place your fingers either behind your knee or on the side of your shin, based on space. Retain your back position and loosen up your shoulders. Remain in position between one to thirteen breaths and switch the sides.

4. Cat and Cow Pose

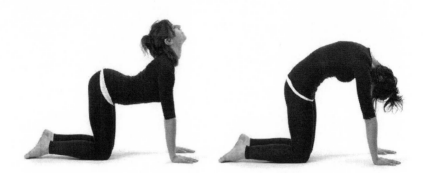

You can expand the hips and the whole body with this easy action.

- Begin on the hands and knees. Lift your chest and tailbone upward while you inhale, and curve your back when you exhale, then push the shoulder blades and pull your head down.
- Stick to the rhythm of your exhaling and inhaling. Sense the muscles on your back and do further movements as you are able.
- Do six to eight sets.

5. Downward Facing Dog

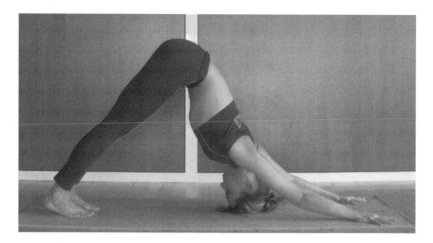

Downward Facing Dog is a great pose to elongate and loosen the whole spine. It also expands the hamstrings and ameliorates back problems.

- Place your toes and palms firmly on the mat and rise into Downward Facing Dog. Begin bent knees, a flat and lengthy back, with the tailbone in the direction of the ceiling. Steadily flatten and stretch out one leg at a time as you take the feet down to the floor.

- Draw the shoulder blades to the spinal column and deliberately attempt to bend them, extending your upper arms outward. Hold for five breaths.

  The lower back protects the entire body, and it's necessary to look after it. Sit still less and move more, elongating and strengthening the back muscles. If you're having chronic discomfort, check with a physician to ensure damaging happens.

10 Yoga Poses for Sciatica Pain Relief

What is sciatica and how can yoga help?

The sciatic nerve begins at the bottom of the back and goes deep through the buttocks and hips and along the legs. Sciatica is induced by the stiffness of the sciatic nerve or relatively low vertebrae discomfort or trauma. Stiff Muscles that are stiff or wounded can also lead to sciatica.

Sciatica pain is a sense of sharpness or a pulsating pain down your leg. You may feel itching, dizziness and swelling. Sciatica is often felt on one side of the body. Sciatica is often nothing than a slight nuisance which causes mild irritation, but it can lead to severe pain.

Cobra pose and Locust pose are essential in improving sciatic signs.

- Reducing the risk of developing backaches
- Improving movement limits
- Reducing the use of pain medications

Let's look at how to use yoga's clinical application to assist in the prevention, soothing and cure of sciatica.

1. Child's Pose (Bal asana)

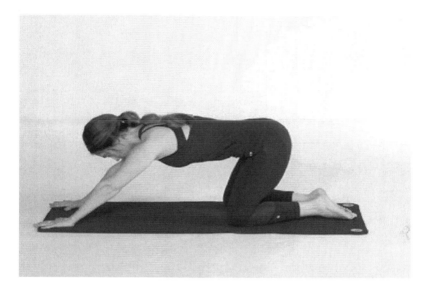

Child's pose is a fantastic way to get your body in rhythm in and relieve stress. It elongates your spine, facilitating stability, including in your hips, thighs and lower back muscles.

- For further help, put a cushion or bolster under your thighs and chest.
- Begin from bent knees and arms. Position your knees together and move your thighs to your heels.
- Stretch out your hands or let them relax along your body.
- Let your torso relax as you fall into your thighs.
- To ease areas of stiffness or emotions, make your breath shallow.
- Keep pose three to five breaths.

2. Downward-Facing Dog

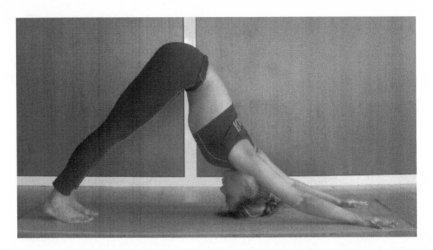

This forward bending position stabilizes the body and relieves tension and stiffness. Downward-Facing Dog encourages resilience throughout your body while correcting imbalances.

- Begin with your knees and arms bent. Push your arms while raising your hips towards the ceiling.
- Lower your head and position the ears to the chest in line with your upper arms or jawline.
- Move your knees down and gently flip the pelvis forward.
- Shift the body into whatever pose feels good.
- Keep this pose up to one minute.

3. Half Moon Pose (Ardha Chandrasana)

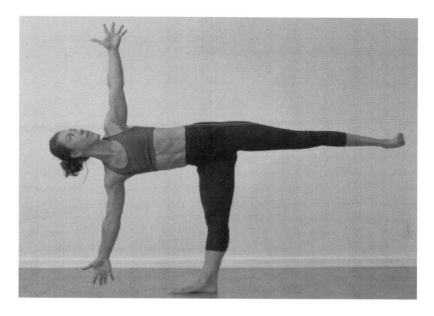

Half Moon pose solidifies your body and helps balance it. It improves flexibility, reduces stress, and stretches the spinal column, glutes, and hips.

Do this posture against a wall. You can put a block under your arm.

- Get into a standing posture with your right foot directly ahead, making a triangle.
- Bend your knee deeper and shift your weight to your right foot.
- Position your left hand on your thigh.
- Move your left foot a few inches forward and the right arm to the ground next to your right foot.

- Raise the left leg parallel to the ground, pushing your left heel.
- Turn your torso and shift your weight to your hip as you stare forward.
- Put your left hand towards the ceiling to go deep and switch your eyes upwards.
- Maintain for one minute.
- Release slowly by bending your right leg and lowering the left leg to the ground, returning to the initial position.
- Perform the movement on the other side.

4. Cobra Pose (Bhujangasana)

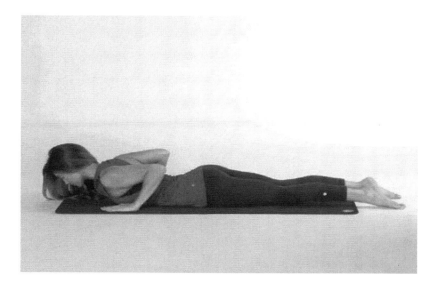

This relaxing posture supports and stretches the, facilitating mobility and flexibility.

- Lie on your chest, shoulders and arms.
- Keep squeezing the elbows into the body.
- Breathe in to lift your head, shoulder, and chest region.
- Hold your elbows slightly bent and your chest open.
- Start engaging the thighs, back muscles, and lower abdomen.
- Hold thirty seconds.
- Relax the pose and repeat one to three times.

5. Locust Pose (Salabhasana)

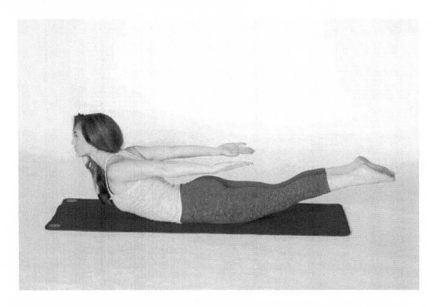

This pose helps boost the spine, glutes, and hips. It strengthens your lower back muscles and core. It also encourages strength and mobility in the thighs.

- Lie on your stomach with your fingertips pulled in at the core of your spine.
- Raise your chest, head, and hands steadily as efficient as possible.
- Position your hands up and apart from your body.
- To go higher, lift both or one leg at a moment.
- Start engaging your lower back muscles, glutes, and abdomen.
- Maintain thirty seconds.

- Start releasing the pose and return to the initial position.
- Pause and breathe for a few minutes, while shifting the hands slowly from side to side.
- Repeat for about one to two times.

6. Knees-to-Chest Pose/Wind-Relieving Pose (Pawanmuktasana)

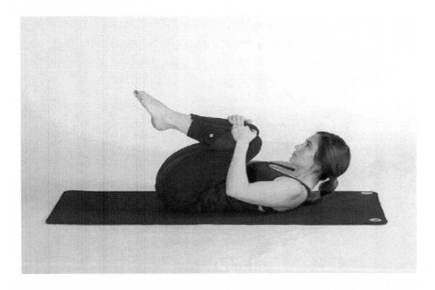

This is an ideal posture to ease lower back stiffness, the buttocks, and glutes. Do one leg at a time for a less severe result.

- Lie down and pull both knees to the chest.
- Bring the ankles and knees together, reaching your arms across your thighs near your shins.
- When your hands meet, interweave your fingers or grasp opposing elbows.
- Raise your head up and move the jawline into your chest to intensify the extension.
- Keep for one minute in this position.

7. Reclined Pigeon Pose (Supta Kapotasana)

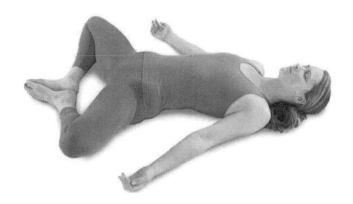

Practicing Pigeon pose on the back assists in supporting the lower back with little stress on the thighs. It extends your glutes and thighs, and also the muscles of the piriformis in the buttocks.

- Lie on your back with your knees bent slightly and your heels towards your thighs.
- Push the right leg and move the right foot to the lower left thigh.
- Remain in place for a profound extension.
- Raise your left foot to go lower and pull your left leg toward your chest.
- Interweave your fingers underneath your left thigh.
- Hold for one minute.
- Repeat on the other side.

8. Bridge Pose (Setu Bandha Sarvangasana)

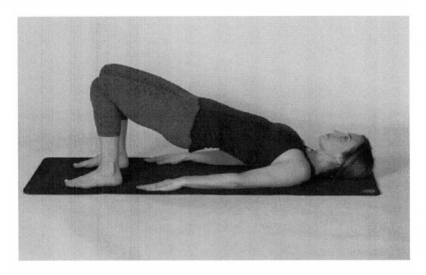

Bridge pose extends the spine, alleviating stiffness, and stress. Its delicately stimulating effect enhances the body's circulatory system. It works your legs, glutes and the core.

- Lie on your back with your knees bent slightly and your heels bent towards your thighs.
- Hold your palms face down beside your body.
- Raise your spinal column from the ground gradually and raise your thighs as best you can.
- To keep in alignment, position a block between your knees or thighs.
- Drop back gradually.
- Maintain the position for one minute at the top.
- Perform again for ten times.
- relax your body as needed.

9. Half Lord of the Fishes Pose (Ardha Matsyendrasana)

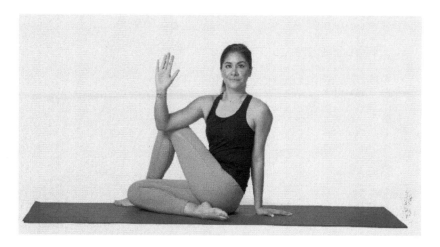

This pose extends the spinal column and elongates it, soothing stress and relieving discomfort. Sense the mobility beginning in your lower back muscles.

- Begin in a sitting position. Place your right foot with your leg forward or left hip in the forward direction.
- Shift your left foot outside your right hip.
- Put your left hand to the ground well behind you and keep your fingers taut.
- Tuck your right hand across your left hip or take it to the outside of your left hip.
- Raise and extend your spinal column with every inhalation.

- Stretch a little more with each breath out to move deeper into the posture.
- Put your head in any position you wish.
- Hold one minute.
- Perform on the other side.

10. Legs-Up-the-Wall Pose (Viparita Karani)

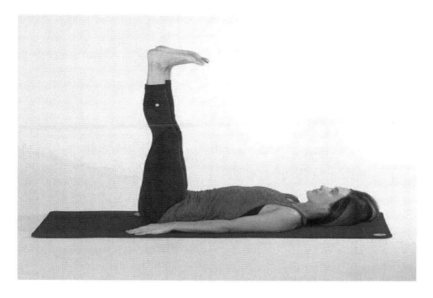

This pose will enable your body to heal, become calm and rebuild tone. Position a pillow or bolster under your thighs to provide comfort.

- Lean against the wall on your right hand.
- Lean back and extend your legs up across the wall, bringing your thighs near the wall as possible.
- Put a cushion below your head, or a folded bedsheet.
- Keep your hands in a relaxed position.
- Let your body relax while you remain calm.
- Hold this posture twenty minutes.

Yoga poses to avoid when you have sciatica

There are a few yoga poses you must ignore once you have sciatica, as they can worsen the symptoms. Recognize your body and what you experience, without attempting to push yourself into any awkward poses.

Experiment and see what actually works for you. Eliminate any pose causing discomfort.

But apart from Downward-Facing Dog, sitting down or standing incorrectly must be averted because they can trigger even more stress in the pelvis and lower spine. From a supine position, you can do forward direction bends (kneeling down, face-up). This allows to shore up your thighs and lower spine.

Although sciatica typically only effects one leg, you may notice that on one side of your body you can do some poses. This is all well. Position pillows in any sitting pose that causes any knee pain. If you have sciatica while pregnant, stop any yoga positions that pinch or stretch the uterus. Stop deep backbends and positions that bring your belly under stress. Use bolsters and to alter poses whenever appropriate.

5 Yoga Poses to Avoid If You Have Piriformis Syndrome

Warrior 3 Pose

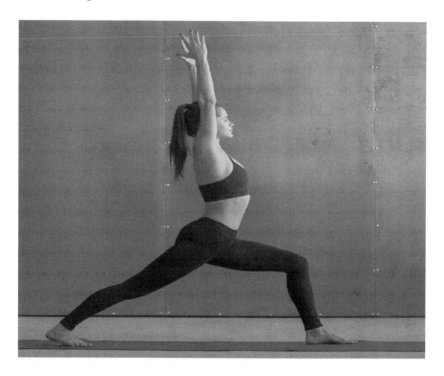

(Remember that putting weight or stretching an injured hip is problematic. I always liked the feel of this pose but felt awful doing it. My glutes and piriformis squirmed las I brought the other leg down. I clearly recall when I could not even move for several minutes. I just stood there patiently, waiting for the discomfort to abate.)

Half Moon Pose

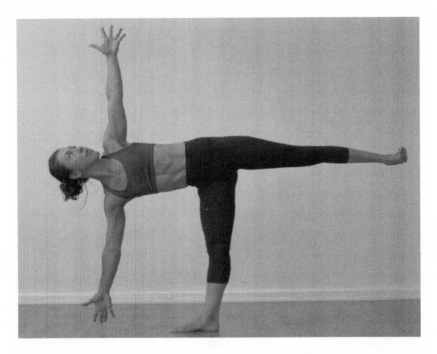

You transition from Warrior 3 when you reach up with your arm. Along with the additional challenge, the alignment component of the pose may ignite more discomfort for some. You 're literally doing a hip abduction, then keeping the glute extended as the pose continues. I work the piriformis muscle to strengthen my thighs when I retain this posture.

Knee to Chest Pose

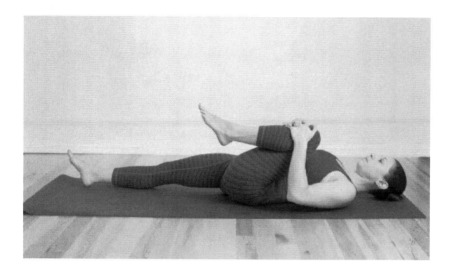

Lie down on a mat and raise one knee all of the way to the chest; it feels good. However, if you let go, the discomfort may pierce the knee and stiffen the outstretched leg. (I couldn't even get up and had to adjust my body gradually which was also unpleasant and then use something to get right back.)

Clearly I wouldn't suggest this workout if get leg pain. There are many other possibilities for the glutes. Moreover, many individuals have very weak glutes and shouldn't even extend them at all.

Reclining Bound Angle Pose

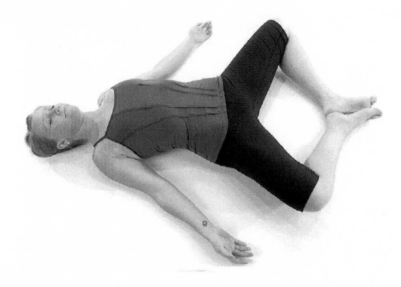

Reclining Bound Angle pose (1): This pose is done by lying flat with your knees outward while trying to bring your feet together. You should sense an extension in the groin area, as your thighs open.

This posture is said to be difficult and detrimental. My issue with it is getting back up. After lying flat on the ground, curving my back, and repositioning my knees, my feet start sinking to open the thighs more (the aim of this workout). It was super traumatic getting out of the pose. I was had terrible groin and glute discomfort attempting to move my thighs. I had to use my arms physically to drag my knees back up, then flip to the mat's edge to get up.

Now, I certainly prefer the pose to the recumbent modification. Rather than lying flat on the floor, lift your spine with a few cushions or do it on the sofa so your thighs can be comfortably positioned. Or attempt this variation of thigh-opening while sitting.

Pigeon Pose

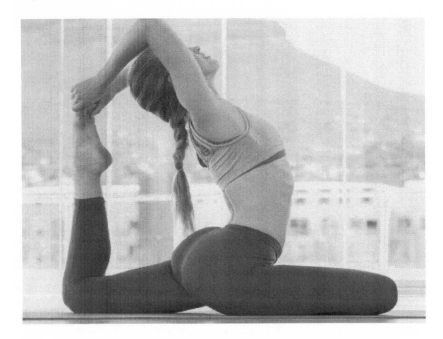

This is a familiar yoga pose that some seventy percent of the time triggers pain. The extension was just too hard for my knees. A better solution is the 90-90degree alternative. I do that all the time as a gentler, simpler variation.

The 4 Best Stretching Exercises to Ease Groin Pain

Certain movements result in groin pain and tight or weak groin muscles (adductors) from groin twists or stretches. The simplest way to manage groin problems is a well-rounded exercise regimen that covers various areas of the body, including past injuries.

Although it is important to consult a professional healthcare or trainer to devise the ideal plan, there are certain prevention steps to avoid groin tightness.

There is reliable, elongating program for a warmup or after exercise. The sequence of activities can be used as an elongating program to cure groin pain and prohibit future groin pulls.

Standing Groin Stretch Exercise

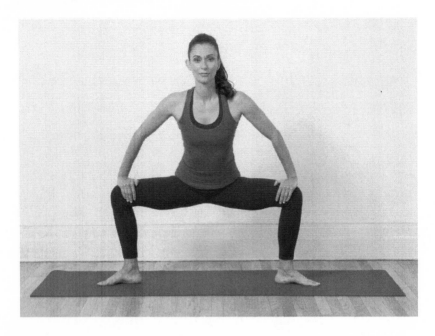

Stand on your legs with bent knees and knees well apart.

Shift your weight towards the left.

Let the left knee curve till over the left foot. You'll feel a slight pull in the right groin.

Retain the position for twenty to thirty seconds.

Repeat the stretching on the same side, then the side 3 times.

Seated Groin Stretch

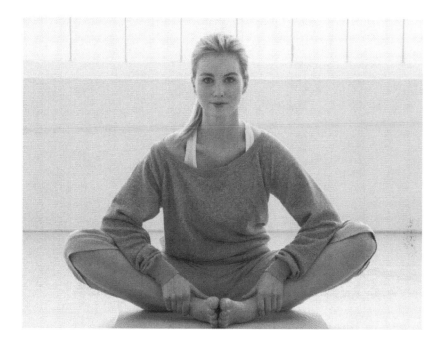

This simple stretch, occasionally called as the stretch of the butterfly, stretches the groin and inner hip.

To get it right:

- Get into a sitting position.
- Place the knees down and bring the sole of your feet together.
- Keep your arms on your feet and your elbows on your knees.
- Let your knees to fall to the floor (no slouching) while maintaining a taut back. You can exert slight pressure on the inner hip by gently rubbing the elbow on the

knees. A squeezing and small discomfort may be felt in the groin. Do not lose your balance and do not exert tremendous effort to stabilize.

- Retain pose for twenty to thirty seconds. Releasing 3 times and repeat again.

- Place the feet closer towards the groin direction to significantly boost the extension.

- By slowly moving forward at the hips, you can get a shallower extension of the hips and back if you're more flexible. Breathe in and lean forward, maintaining the back flat, and let your chest fall as near to the ground as you can.

Squatting Groin Stretch

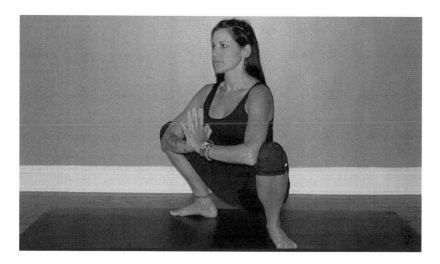

This is a bit of a more complex groin extension that amplifies the exercise on both at once

- Stand with feet apart, toes pointed outward.
- Squat at a 90-degree angle till your knees are above your ankles.
- Put your palms on top of your inner thighs and move your thighs steadily outwards. In both legs you will feel an extension in the groin muscles.
- Hold for twenty to thirty seconds, rest and repeat again three times.

Hip Opener and Groin Stretch

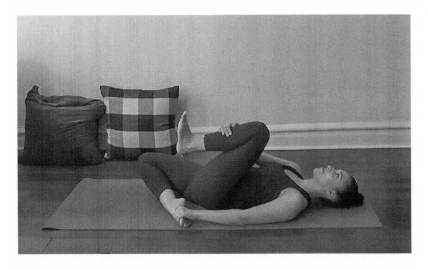

This workout increases the flexibility of the hips, groin and lower spine muscles.

- Start in a forward thrust pose on the floor and push your left knee to the floor.
- Put your right elbow along the inside of your right knee.
- Simply push your right elbow to your right knee and reposition your upper body to the left.
- Your left arm in place, you will sense a gentle extension in your back muscles and in the right groin.
- Hold the stretch, relax it and perform it on the other leg for around twenty to thirty seconds.

This stretch may be modified depending on your own anatomy, adaptability, and constraints. If you are suffering from knee pain, be careful to hold your forward knee over or just behind your ankle and not above the ankle.

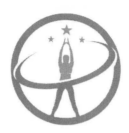

Chapter 7:
Soreness After Yoga

It is no wonder that you feel a little achy after yoga — particularly if you are just getting back into it or doing postures you typically do not do it. After all, the reason a regular yoga practice feels so great is because it can profoundly stretch those muscles you do not have access to in your everyday life.

"You may feel your muscles are strong, but some yoga poses will still stretch them out in unexpected ways," say yoga experts. "Muscles also will get sore because they have been overused."

The soreness you may feel after yoga is called (DOMS) acronymfor delayed onset muscle soreness, which typically occurs within 12-48 hours of exercising. The intensity of soreness you might experience depends on the style, how vigorously you are doing it, and how often. as well as the condition of your individual body. And even though you are experienced in your training, there is a fair chance that you will still feel sore. Yoga is typically a low-impact workout. but it can put great strain on your muscles.

Yoga is packed with eccentric contractions that trigger muscular and fascial tissue microscopic injury. Expert says that "our bodies send these micro-tears an inflammatory response and this induces muscle soreness."

Yet this muscle soreness turns out to be a positive thing. "You'll be experiencing muscle development and better results until your muscles heal," says yoga experts, eventually making you stronger. If the soreness is very uncomfortable after yoga, of course, see a doctor. However, there are plenty of clever tricks you can use to relieve the discomfort of the run-of-the-mill soreness with minimal pain.

Hydrate, then hydrate a little more

Drink water but not sports drinks, say yoga experts. We want to help raise our blood flow so that this fluid can be more efficiently circulated to the tissues so energy is transferred, cells are healed and metabolic waste flushes out. This is the way hydration occurs.

DO get plenty of sleep

Your body cannot "gear down" without sleep; it needs to rest to allow the parasympathetic nervous system (digest-and-rest mode) to be in control. "The neuroendocrine system won't prepare the body and tissues for recovery and relaxation without a proper sleep."

DON'T down caffeine and energy supplements

According to experts, unless you are an ultra-endurance performer, you are not likely to deplete your body so much that you need caffeine, energy drinks or supplements. "It adds more needless calories and other substances to a body that only requires gentle movement, hydration and rest."

DO exercise—gently

Exercising is the safest way after meditation to alleviate soreness. In addition, research shows performing the same muscle movements and sequences you did before you felt sore

— in a less extreme way — may help alleviate muscle spasms, allowing muscles, connective tissue and joints to recover a greater range of movement.

Use a foam roller

Right after working out, 20 minutes of foam rolling will alleviate tenderness — even though it causes some discomfort. Take it easy and be gentle; you do not want to inflict so much damage that it really makes your soreness worse.

DO eat a balanced meal

Make sure your snack or meal after exercise contains protein that strengthens and develops muscle, as well as carbohydrates, which will also speed up recovery.

DON'T take anti-inflammatory drugs

It that sound like a smart idea to take aspirin to take the edge off your soreness after exercise, but this is not the key to recovery. "Inflammation is how the body reacts to an injury of some sort." To heal any damaged tissue properly, you must have inflammation. When you cut off the inflammation with a drug you inhibit the normal healing mechanisms of your body.

DO take a hot bath

This not only feels fantastic, but it also helps activate the parasympathetic nervous system to relieve stress and allow the body to attain a healing state.

DO stretch

And if you stretch, make sure to go through all the motion planes. This should improve movement and motion range while also avoiding chronic stress and pain.

DON'T do intense stretching

Long, tense stretches, or excessive stretching sore muscles do more damage than good. "The tissues are already slightly weakened and working on healing." When you over-stretch the muscles and affect their fluids, you can decrease their healing ability and even damage them.

DO continue to practice yoga, gently

Some of the very best ways to deal with soreness after yoga is to do more yoga. "Concentrate on the places suffering and slowly strive to alleviate pain and tightness." Becoming lazy because of soreness is a very poor answer to your soreness, and the next time you practice yoga will probably leave you in much more pain.

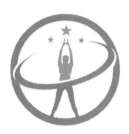

Chapter 8:
Discover How Yoga Poses and Meditation can Improve Your Anatomy

If you are a committed yoga practitioner, you have probably found some benefit from yoga — perhaps sleeping better, getting fewer cold, or just feeling more confident and relaxed. And if you have ever tried to convince a newbie about the advantages of yoga, you should mention that it enhances prana flow or brings energy.

38 Ways Yoga Improves Anatomy

My experience has encouraged me to pore over the research studies I have collected to discuss how yoga can both avoid and help you recover from disease.

1. Improves flexibility

One of the first and most noticeable advantages of yoga is improved flexibility. You will not touch your feet or do a backbend during your first lesson. But if you stick to it, you could experience a progressive loosening, and seemingly impossible poses gradually become feasible. You will probably also find that pains and aches begin to vanish. This is no coincidence. Due to the poor alignment of the thighs and shinbones, tight hips can strain the knee joints. Some tight muscles cause a flattening of the lumbar spine that can lead to back pain. And muscle and connective tissue inflexibility, fascia and ligaments may add to poor posture.

2. Builds muscle strength

Healthy muscles do much more than look toned. They also defend against diseases such as arthritis and back pain and help avoid falls in the elderly. And when yoga creates energy, you can balance all this with greater flexibility. If you just join a gym and lift weights, at the cost of flexibility, you may not be gaining what you need.

3. Perfects your posture

Your head is like a rubber ball — heavy, big, and round. If it is directly over an upright spine, the neck and back muscles require much less effort to sustain it. However, push it forward several inches and you start straining those muscles. Keep the forward-leaning bowling ball up for eight or twelve hours a day and no surprise at however tired you are. This may not be your only fatigue problem. Bad posture can cause problems with your back, neck, and other muscles and joints. As you slump, the body may adjust by straightening your neck and lower back with the usual inward curve. This can cause backbone strain and painful degenerative arthritis.

4. Protects cartilage and broken joint

When you do yoga, every time you use a full range of movement in the joints. This helps avoid degenerative arthritis or reduces disability by using cartilage areas not usually exercised. Joint cartilage is like a sponge; it only absorbs nutrients when its fluid has been drained out, so it can soak up a new supply. Without proper support, neglected cartilage areas can gradually wear down, showing the inner bone like worn-out brake pads.

5. Protects your spine

Shock absorbers between the vertebrae prevent pinch nerves. Exercise is way to receive nutrients. When you practice well-balanced asana with enough forward bends, backbends, and twists you help to maintain your discs supple.

6. Improves bone health

It is well known that weight-bearing exercise improves the bones and helps prevent osteoporosis. Many Yoga postures allow you to hold your own weight. Our arm bones may strengthen, which is of value for those especially sensitive to osteoporotic fractures. Perform poses like Upward and Downward-Facing Dog. In an experimental study conducted at California State University in Los Angeles, yoga practice was shown to increase bone density in the vertebrae. Yoga's ability to reduce stress hormone cortisol levels may help maintain bone calcium.

7. Increases blood flow

Yoga makes for better blood flow. More importantly, the relaxation practices you learn in yoga, particularly in your hands and feet, can improve circulation. Yoga also gives the cells more oxygen, helping them to function better overall. It is thought that twisting poses move venous blood out of the internal organs and permit oxygenated blood to flow in until the twist is released. Inverted poses, such as Handstand, standing Headstand, and Shoulder stand enable venous blood from the legs and pelvis to stream back to the heart, where it can be transferred to the lungs for fresh oxygenation.

This will help if heart or kidney issues cause swelling in your legs. Hemoglobin and red blood cells level improve through Yoga and a good oxygen supply to the tissues. And its thins the blood by making platelets less sticky and reducing the amount of proteins that cause clots. This can lead to a decline in heart attacks and strokes as these killers also cause blood clots.

8. Drain your lymph nodes and improve immunity

Lymph drainage (a viscous fluid rich in immune cells) can increase as you compress and extend muscles, shift organs, and come in and out yoga poses. This allows the lymphatic system to fight disease, cancer cells are killed, and cellular working radioactive waste products are disposed of.

9. Raises the heart rate

Heart failure risk may be reduced as you relieve stress if your heart rate regularly reaches the aerobic zone. And if you practice daily, or take flow or Ashtanga classes, it can lift the heart rate into the aerobic zone, while not all types of yoga are aerobic. Also, yoga exercises enhance cardiovascular fitness.

Studies show that yoga practice reduces the heart rate at rest, improves stamina and can improve daily oxygen consumption during exercise — all manifestations of enhanced aerobic fitness. One research study found subjects taught only pranayama were able to do more exercises with less oxygen.

10. Drops blood pressure

Whether you have high blood pressure or not, you may be benefiting from yoga. Two studies of people with hypertension published in the British medical journal, The Lancet, compared Savasana (Corpse pose) results with sitting on a couch. After three months, Savasana was associated with a fifteen-point decrease in diastolic blood pressure and a twenty-six-point decrease in systolic blood pressure; the greater the decrease, the higher the initial blood pressure.

11. Loads up the adrenal glands

Your cortisol levels can be lowered by yoga. Think about it. Usually, the adrenal glands release cortisol in response to an intense crisis that temporarily improves immune function. When the cortisol levels remain high after the crisis, the immune system may be weakened. Temporary cortisol increases help improve long-term memory, but excessively elevated levels impair memory and can result in permanent brain changes.

In addition, excessive cortisol has been associated with severe depression, osteoporosis (that eliminates calcium and other bone minerals and interferes with laying fresh bone), insulin resistance and high blood pressure. High levels of cortisol in rats result in what scientists call food-seeking behavior (causing you to eat when frustrated, angry or stressed). The body takes these additional calories and distributes them in the abdomen as fat, leading to weight gain, diabetes risk and a possible heart attack.

12. Makes you happier

One study found that daily yoga practice decreased depression and contributed to a substantial increase in serotonin levels and a decrease in monoamine oxidase (the enzyme that breaks down neurotransmitters) levels as well as levels of cortisol. It was found that the left prefrontal cortex displayed increased activation in meditators, a result associated with higher satisfaction rates and improved immune function. In committed, long-term practitioners, more drastic left-hand activation has been found.

13. Provides a healthy lifestyle

Run more, eat less. On all sides yoga can be of benefit. Daily exercise will get you moving and burn calories, and your practice's spiritual and emotional nature will motivate you to tackle any eating and weight issues at a deeper level. Yoga will also inspire you to be a more conscious consumer.

14. Lowers blood sugar

Yoga reduces blood sugar and LDL (bad) cholesterol and raises cholesterol in HDL (good). Yoga has been shown for those with diabetes to reduce blood sugar in many ways by reducing cortisol and adrenaline levels, promoting weight loss and increasing sensitivity to the effects of insulin. As our blood sugar levels goes up, the risk of diabetic complications rise, including kidney failure, heart attack, and blindness.

15. Focus may help you

Studies have found that the daily practice of yoga enhances balance, time of response, memory, as well as IQ scores. People who follow Transcendental Meditation have the ability to solve problems and learn and recall information — probably because they are less overwhelmed by their emotions, which play like an endless tape loop over and over again.

16. Relaxes your system

You may become relaxed by yoga and can calm your breathing and concentrate on current circumstances, shifting the balance from the sympathetic nervous system towards the parasympathetic nervous system. The latter is relaxing and restorative; it reduces breathing and heart rate, lowers blood pressure, and raises blood pressure to the intestines and reproductive organs.

17. Improves equilibrium

Regular yoga practice improves the sense of touch (whatever the body is doing and where it is) and promotes equilibrium. People with poor posture or a habit of dysfunctional motion typically have impaired proprioception, which also relates to knee problems and back pain. Better equilibrium may mean fewer falls. This translates into greater freedom and delayed entry to a nursing home for the aged, or never accessing one at all. For the rest of us, postures like Tree pose will help us feel steady on the ground.

18. Maintains your nervous system

Some experienced yogis can exercise remarkable control of their bodies, some of which are mediated by the nervous system. Scientists have been studying yogis who trigger irregular heart rhythms, produce unique brainwave patterns, and increase the temperature of their hands by fifteen degree (F) when using a meditation technique. Yoga can be used if you want to get pregnant or relax when having trouble sleeping. You will learn how to increase blood flow to your pelvis.

19. Releases tension in your limbs

Do you ever find grabbing the telephone or a steering wheel with a tight grip or clenching your face while looking at a computer screen? These unintentional habits can lead to chronic strain, muscle weakness and pain in your arms, wrists, neck, shoulders, and face, which increase stress and worsen mood. As we practice yoga, we begin to note that we keep stress, perhaps in the head, tongue, or face and neck muscles. You might relieve some stress in the tongue and the eyes if you just tune in. It takes years of practice to relax larger muscles like the trapezius, quadriceps, and buttocks.

20. Helps you sleep deeper

Stimulation is great unless it stimulates the nervous system too much. Yoga will alleviate the hustle and bustle of daily life. Restorative asana, yoga nidra (a form of directed relaxation), pranayama, Savasana, and meditation promote pratyahara, a turning of the senses inward, which provides the nervous system with much-needed downtime. Studies say that another byproduct of daily yoga practice is improved sleep — which means you will be less exhausted and depressed, also less likely to have accidents.

21. Functionality of the immune system increases

The immune system strengthens by doing Asana and pranayama, but in this area, meditation has so far been the best help. It tends to have a positive effect on immune system functioning, improving it when needed (e.g. raising antibody levels in regard to a vaccine) and reducing it when required (e.g. minimizing an overly aggressive immune function in an autoimmune disease such as psoriasis).

22. Gives your lungs room to breathe

Yogis take more intense breaths that are both relaxing and more effective. A 1998 study published in The Lancet demonstrated a yogic procedure known as complete respiration for people with lung problems due to congestive heart failure. Their average respiratory rate dropped from 13.4 breathes per minute to 7.6 after one month. Meanwhile their potential for exercise improved dramatically, as did their blood oxygen saturation. Additionally, yoga has been shown to enhance various lung functions, including optimum breath volume and exhalation capacity.

Yoga also encourages breathing through the nose, cleansing the air and warming it up (cold, dry air is more likely to cause an asthma attack in susceptible people). It humidifies it, eliminating pollen, dirt, and other stuff you would rather not allow into your lungs.

23. Prevents IBS and other digestive problems

Irritable bowel syndrome, ulcers, and constipation may be aggravated by stress. And if you worry less, then you are going to suffer less. As with any physical activity, yoga can relieve constipation — and potentially minimize the risk of colon cancer — because shifting the body enables the quicker movement of food and waste products in the intestines. And while it has not been tested scientifically, yogis claim that rotating positions can be helpful in getting waste moving around the body.

24. Gives you peace of mind

Yoga washes away disturbances of thought. In other words, it slows down the mental loops that can trigger stress, such as disappointment, guilt, frustration, fear, and desire. Since stress is involved in so many health issues — from migraines and insomnia to lupus, eczema, MS, and heart attacks, and high blood pressure — if you are trying to relax your mind, you are likely to live longer and safer.

25. Increases your self-esteem

Most of us have chronically poor self-esteem. When you treat this negatively — take medications, work too hard, overeat, sleep around — you may be physically, emotionally, and morally paying the price for poorer health. If you take an active approach and practice yoga, you know that you are worthy, or as yogic philosophy says, you are a representation of the Divine, initially in fleeting glimpses and later from more prolonged views.

When you frequently exercise with the goal of self-examination and improvement — not just as a replacement for an aerobics class — you can reach another part of yourself. You will experience feelings of appreciation, empathy, and acceptance, as well as a sense that something bigger is your responsibility.

26. Relax the pain

Asana, meditation, or a combination of both decreased pain in people with fibromyalgia, arthritis, carpal tunnel syndrome, back pain, and other severe conditions. Yoga also soothes discomfort. You are more likely to be healthy when you relieve pain, your mood improves, but you do not need that much medicine.

27. Gives you inner strength

Yoga will help you make positive improvements, potentially its greatest asset. Tapas is the Sanskrit word for heat, to be the fire, the discipline which fuels the practice of yoga and builds up daily practice. You should apply the tapas to the rest of your life to overcome boredom and change unhealthy behaviors. You may find that you start eating healthier, exercising more, or actually stopping smoking after years of unsuccessful attempts, without making any real effort.

28. Connects you with guidance

Great yoga instructors can do wonders for health. Exceptional ones do something other than lead you through the postures. You can adjust your posture, gauge if you should go further into a pose or back off. Yoga delivers compassionate hard truths, helps calm the body and mind, and helps you develop and customize your practice. A positive partnership with a teacher helps to improve wellbeing.

29. Helps keep you drugs free

If your cabinet of medications looks like a pharmacy, then the time has come to try yoga. Studies have shown that people with high blood pressure, asthma, diabetes (also known as adult-onset diabetes), and obsessive-compulsive disorder can practice yoga to make it easier for them to minimize their drug dosage of and even get them off entirely. You would spend less money on medications, and you are less likely to suffer side effects or adverse reactions from medications.

30. Builds knowledge for improvement

Yoga builds consciousness. The more you are conscious, the simpler it is to relieve yourself of negative emotions such as rage. Studies show that persistent rage and aggression are as closely related as smoking, diabetes, and elevated cholesterol to heart attacks. Yoga tends to alleviate frustration by increasing compassion and an interconnection between emotions while relaxing the nervous system and mind. It also increases the ability to step back from life's drama, to stay calm in the face of negative news or disturbing happenings. You can always respond rapidly when you want to—and there's proof that yoga increases response time—but you may take a half second to select a more careful method, ultimately reducing your and others' suffering.

31. Benefits your relationships

Love cannot overcome anything but in healing it will definitely help. Repeatedly maintaining the emotional support of family, friends, and society has been shown to enhance health and healing. The daily practice of yoga helps cultivate friendliness, humility, and greater equanimity. Along with the focus of yogic philosophy on preventing harm to others, speaking the truth and only taking what you need, this should strengthen many of your relationships.

32. Uses sounds to clear the sinuses

Pranayama, asana, and meditation are the basics of yoga used to improve health. It appears to prolong exhalation, thus changing balance towards the parasympathetic nervous system. Chanting can be an especially powerful physical and emotional activity when performed. A recent study indicates that humming sounds – like those produced when singing Om – open the sinuses and promote drainage.

33. Guides your body's healing in your mind's eye

You can alter your body if you visualize a picture in your mind's eye, as you would do in yoga nidra and other practices. Several studies have shown that supervised imagery lowered postoperative pain, decreased headache frequency, and enhanced quality of life for cancer and HIV sufferers.

34. Held allergies and viruses in place

Kriyas are another component of yoga, as calming activities. They involve everything from short breathing exercises to the elaboration of internal intestinal cleansings. Jala neti, which requires a soft lavage of the nasal passages with salt water, removes viruses and pollen from the nose, stops mucus from building up, and helps clear the sinuses.

35. Helps you serve others

The central aspect of yogic philosophy is yoga karma. Even though you may not be able to support others, when you do, you will improve your health. Serving others may bring value to your life and your struggle will appear so difficult when you see what others are dealing with.

36. Encourages self-care

Most patients of traditional medicine are passive treatment receivers. In Yoga, what matters is what you do for yourself. Yoga provides the tools to improve the first time you practice; at the start, you well might start feeling better. Note that the more you indulge in exercise, the more you gain. This results in three things for your own care: you find that your engagement gives you the power to improve and knowing that you can improve offers hope. And hope can be healing itself.

37. Supports your connective tissue

You have already found similarities in the ways Yoga enhances health. That is because they are tightly intertwined. Shift your posture and adjust your way of breathing. Change your respiration and improve your nervous system. Connecting everything is one of the great lessons of yoga — your hipbone to your anklebone, you to your friends, you to the universe. This connection is vital in understanding yoga. At the same time, this holistic approach taps into several mechanisms that have additional and even multiplicative effects. This is the most powerful way to treat yoga.

38. Uses the placebo effect to modify

You have to believe you will get better. Unfortunately, a lot of mainstream scientists assume it does not matter if something succeeds by the placebo effect. But most people just want to feel better, so if repeating a mantra — like you might do it at the beginning or end of a yoga session, during a meditation, or during the day — facilitates recovery, even if it's only a placebo effect.

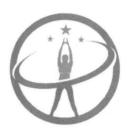

Chapter 9:
How to Meditate

The key purpose of meditative practice is to move the brain's attention away from the frantic concerns of daily life, such as stresses regarding work, relationships, investments, or even the day's "to-do list." Specific meditation experience is needed to impart potential benefits to the patients appropriately and honestly. Meditation means preparing your mind to remain in the moment, as there is real happiness in the current situation.

There are three main types of meditative observations: concentrative, verbal, and motion. Descriptions of therapy include designing or sketching, practicing in the garden, looking at the water, interacting with your cat, newspapering, telling your kid how to learn a skill, openly listening to your favorite music etc. Other types of meditation contain tai chi and yoga that include relaxation practice with rehearsed moves. These traditional ways of meditation nourish the brain after stressful emotions and place the brain in a calm and peaceful condition in accordance with physical movements through careful ventilation. Imaginative therapy means finding an expression for the artistic side as claimed by neurologists for the cerebral hemisphere.

Introduction

After studying and absorbing the academic debate on the various health advantages related to meditation, it is very easy for the active physician to literally advise patients to "try to meditate." Therefore, when a physician who has not himself studied meditation offers advice — no wonder how genuine, well-meaning, or scientifically acceptable — the suggestion is there.

To convey adequately and honestly the effects that you want a particular patient to receive for his or her specific needs, prior familiarity with meditation is needed, and it is difficult to express this knowledge with certainty until you "learn" how the meditation technique has influenced your own mental and physical health. When you talk with the credibility of professional knowledge regarding your "meditation order," and actively advise your patients while you give detailed guidance on how to meditate, it will incredibly unlikely for your patients not to take on the passion underlying your suggestion, making the more likely to be followed.

Does not every doctor after all wish his or her patients to take advice so they can improve health? Training to meditate and beginning a daily meditation routine are essential means of strengthening the life of patients and physicians too. The key purpose of the meditative practice is to move the mind away from the hassles and routine of daily life. There are numerous ways or strategies to consider

What is meditation?

Meditation means attempting to prepare your mind to remain in the current moment, as there is real happiness in the present. Potential views (what can / could / will occur that result in dread or anxiousness) or previous memories (what did or could have did, resulting in sorrow, disappointment, rage, or jealousy) keep one from experiencing the current calm. Being completely centered on the current moment means you don't care about the past or the future as they have been released from the negative feelings (stress) for as the mediation process lasts.

EXAMPLES OF MEDITATION

• Can you imagine an operation where you neglect to keep track of time completely? When you center your mind and you say, "I don't know where the time has gone?" Explanations could be doing artwork or designing, mowing the lawn, sunning at the beach, playing with your cat, writing emails, showing your kid how to play basketball, comfortably listening to your favorite songs, etc. I realized that when doing treatments in the operating theater, I really concentrated so that my procedures became actual meditations.

• Each of these conditions are meditative moments since there are no previous or expected ideas; the brain is only aware of the current moment.

• As you focus on the experience(s) of your life and that you lost track of time, you may remember that you also lost track of what caused you pain, whether from a dysfunctional friendship, a debilitating condition, or the sorrow that occurs with disappointment or death.

CATEGORIES OF MEDITATION

If you have a passion or any kind of exercise to indulge in on a routine basis that allows you to lose track of time count yourself one of the fortunate. The rest of us (most people in the world) have to allocates time on their calendars for a quiet-mind meditation. As noted in above details, these interactions can be subdivided into three major categories:

- Concentrative
- Movement
- Expressive

These three methods of meditation have been practiced in various tradition and religions for decades. I will provide descriptions for every group, and will recommend that you play with them all so you have sufficient knowledge to understand what you prefer most (as the foundation of your daily meditation exercise) and also to know how to better communicate with patients.

How to Meditate

- First, arranging time for inner contemplation is paramount.
- We all have busy schedules and with the right mindset, but sometimes life has a cost of not planning. (Mostly people lack the ability to allay this challenge until they stick to a specific schedule.)
- So, training in meditation means having time on a regular basis. The great news here is that it does not take a lot of time. A newcomer can do only a few minutes a day, gradually hitting 20 to 30 minutes a day

as the advantages become apparent as a very valuable part of the day.

CONCENTRATIVE TECHNIQUES

- First, I will address exact strategies as these factors are defined, learned and most frequently used.

- Both include intense attention and concentrating the mind actively on something important. They involve looking at a dancing candle flame, saying a phrase (or mantra) to yourself repeatedly (such as harmony, happiness, or God), or simply listening to your heart. The purpose is to focus and simply ignore other ideas that inevitably will pop up into your brain.

- The trick is to let certain emotions come forth and then let them go while not getting wrapped up in them.

Tips for Applying the Concentrative Techniques

- Do not think of an unfortunate situation and get choked up. You don't want to start getting upset or wounded again, while plotting your retaliation. That is not a meditative practice, but acts as an example of how a perception about a traumatic event is granted extra control by the feelings behind it as well as the remembered desire for vengeance.

- Instead of feeling this way, do your hardest to acknowledge that this is a scenario taking place, and do your best to concentrate your mind on the flame, etc. and not get lost in past drama. This can be hard to do at first, but can surely be achieved with repetition - while seldom to full excellence except by yogis or monks.

- When you need evidence of the effectiveness of these methods, just ask a successful meditator, who would certainly share his or her inspirational stories and the problems that never went away entirely.

Positioning

- It is necessary to stand correctly until you begin, which suggests you should sit easily and not lie down.

- It is good to sit in a chair with your feet on the ground. Sitting on the floor works, even without a pad, but strive to keep your back as tight as you can without discomfort.

- Tight clothes will disturb you, and your shoes must be off.

- For active and authentic meditation, a peaceful place is ideal as is good weather.

- Many daily meditators want to find a private place to stay focused and they gain from sitting across from items with a specific significance like images of beloved ones, holy artifacts, or quartz (amethyst is said to promote meditation).

- Although attempting to attain such an "ideal" environment is ideal, one of the miracles of meditation is that it can work anywhere, including under the cruelest of circumstances. Even some practitioners have had successful meditations lying on the ground outside within the chaotic mess of a refugee camp.

Quieting the Mind

- The final and key step in preparation for a calm, guided meditation is to execute a strategy that will allow the brain to remain quiet.
- After getting relaxed (as mentioned above), simply take your hand and keep the core of your palm about 3 to 4 inches away from the spot on your forehead at the top of and in the center of your eyebrows above the nose.
- Close your eyes and tilt your hand to create the shape of a circle in the middle of your palm the size of a quarter. Turn your hand to the side, so if you faced an observer, your head would turn in that direction.
- If you slowly expand the circle width when you push your hand, this is not a problem. People derive various feelings from this, such as a sense of heat flowing from

their hands to their foreheads, so it allows the brain to be still.

- It's time to begin concentrating on the item chosen for your meditation (repeating a prayer, looking at a candle, saying a word or phrase or focusing on the breath). Feel your mind has calmed down a little indicates you aren't paying heed to any ideas arising.

FOCUS ON THE BREATH

- Concentrate on breathing is the common concentrative type of meditation.

- This is completely flexible as there is no need for materials (like a candle) and it can be achieved anywhere.

- Simply concentrating on your breathing as it goes in and out of the lungs is the direction for this practice.

- Remember to inhale through your nose and exhale through your mouth (do not panic if your nose is stuffed). Be mindful of the air that goes in and out.

- By holding your breathing focused, you are stopping other ideas from getting into your mind. If they do, just let them go and get back to focus on breathing.

- Seek to do this for a minute or two when you begin first, then carry on longer as you can.

VARIATIONS ON A THEME

- This simplest script has many versions. What you find soothing can be achieved in solitude or with music.

- If you catch your attention shifting to the music away from your breath, let it occur — it is just an alternative way to meditate.

- By incorporating the mental exercise of recalling a word or phrase in your head in sync with your breath, you can regulate your mind. An illustration would be the term "warm belly" - focusing on the word "warm" at the inhale and "belly" at the exhale.

- Another method to organize the meditative cycle is to go through a predetermined sequence of thoughts until initiating the concentrative portion of the practice (in this case on the breath) after feeling relaxed and doing the hand movements mentioned.

An illustration is the thinking process that I actually use on a regular basis, which I provide here for you to use or change to your liking. I am not sharing this with you because I want you to think a particular way but because you may find it helpful. Before beginning my concentrative meditation, this style of thinking calms my brain by taking my stressful feelings a way so they are less likely to interfere with my meditation.

Expressing Gratitude

- I start each of my meditations explicitly by voicing appreciation for all that I have in my lifetime, both the good and the negative.

- This helps me become hope about the obstacles that I might face, allowing me to minimize the stress that accompany difficult situations, even if ever so marginally.

- Then I seek to get to a point of relaxation where I strive to make myself aware that there will be circumstances in my life that I cannot fully comprehend or influence. I no longer lament, "Why me?" When life gets tough, it allows me to embrace the facts of the situation and absorbs a great deal of my emotional strength, helping me to concentrate on the search for answers.

- This is the routine I practice each morning before beginning the concentrative part, clearing my brain and preparing me for a much more successful, deeper, and intense meditation.

SETTLING INTO THE MEDITATIVE MOMENT

- When sitting and concentrating become challenging, you could be better off first doing a meditation on an action.

- You should violently rock your arms or dance all over the room (in tribal, ballroom, modern or ethnic fashion) to the blaring music you absolutely love. It is usually better achieved with nobody present (you might feel self-conscious that you look odd to an outsider). How do you look 5 minutes later? If you want to move on, do so.

- Thereafter, try to maintain your breathing steady for the next few minutes. Do not be disappointed if feelings show up when you shake or dance. This is not an unusual phenomenon, particularly if you have feelings that have not been expressed and lie dormant.

- Intense activity is a good way to go through strong feelings. If this strategy puts out strong feelings that impact you all day long, talking with a therapist may dilute the mental pain.

- Eventually, meditations on personal struggles are a perfect alternative for those trapped in their life, either spiritually or otherwise.

Movement Meditation through Martial Arts

- A description of action therapy is deficient without discussing yoga, tai chi, qigong, and other martial arts that are not only a practice but also a lifestyle in their natural form.

- All of them are traditional practices that integrate regulating thought (mainly through concentrating on breathing) with action (through poses or precisely rehearsed routines) to maintain a balance between body and brain.

- Regarding a couple of these methods, I highly advise all professionals to take an instructional class to see if one is good for you; it will also help you illustrate it to your client. Participation in tai chi combines breathing practice with rehearsed motions.

- A yoga instructor can help purify the brain of stressful emotions and place the mind in a calm and peaceful condition in accordance with physical movements generated by sufficient air.

EXPRESSIVE MEDICATION: CREATING AN OUTLET FOR MEDITATING

- The final meditation type, expressionistic meditation, includes providing an outlet for the expression of your creative side.

- Methods include journaling, painting, or just interacting with rocks - small stones and sticks - encouraging the hands to make anything they want while listening to soothing music and concentrating entirely on the task at hand.

- The approach of journaling is to take personal time and write truthfully and frankly about how you think and behave on every subject that comes up.

- Some organize this by writing the key things of the day and the related emotions and thoughts. Some write about a single subject, like learning about all the problems of a serious illness on a regular basis.

- Most people find that they receive useful insights into their condition when they write just what they think or believe without allowing their egos get in the way (by analyzing their spelling or determining that a subject is off boundaries). They find that they become less anxious and more comfortable.

Conclusions

A significant final point is that this section was intended to relay knowledge on how to meditate at an elementary level, as mentioned in the original description. It was necessary to divulge details that have formerly been kept confidential or described in complex ways. It is now condensed and comprehensible. I decided to teach meditation in a way that anyone could accept and appreciate, without the cultural or spiritual overtones that can act as a barrier. Although this technique took clinical training, it has changed the lives of thousands of people by practicing meditation in this purely secular, simple, and realistic manner. It is my firm conviction that those who desire to study and understand the mystical and metaphysical effects of meditation will be guided to what they truly seek and ultimately discover.

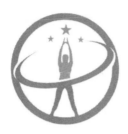

Chapter 10:
How to Use Meditation
to Manage Chronic Pain

rbitrary categories and removing dialogue, I learn, from my own personal experience, of the metaphysical elements of a meditation exercise.

1. The pain is not all in your head

Let us begin by discussing one of the main obstacles for those deciding either to continue using chronic illness meditation. Many people with chronic pain believe that others do not understand the truth of their suffering, so they deny or minimize it. The belief that therapy will help us with our pain is another way to saying that all our suffering is in our minds.

The solution to this common assumption is to recognize that it does not mean that it cannot impact real suffering simply because meditation requires concentration of mind. I taught yoga to people suffering from surgery pain to see the benefit. That is all in their brains, no one can know! Additionally, studies have demonstrated that meditators even with socially mediated pain have greater pain levels than non-meditators.

To recap, being angry when someone questions the truth of your physical suffering is excusable. At the very same time, therapy can help with all types of pain, either physical, mental or a mixture of the two.

2. The paradox of paying attention

The final activity we want to do while in discomfort is to give it our all. Cognitive therapy for people dealing with pain highlights different forms of relaxation before meditation enters the scene. Mindfulness means becoming more conscious, more responsive and not more depressed. Mind experiments have found that the pain-sensing areas of the mind light up as qualified meditators pay more attention to unpleasant stimuli. The parts of the mind responsible for pain-related discomfort are less involved.

It is not only the level of concentration that counts, but the level of attention as well. Chronic pain patients often cultivate a form of focus that is overly vigilant. They may be extremely reactive in their discomfort to a small change. This may not serve to alleviate their discomfort and may render it worse. The kind of concentration that we develop in the practice of meditation is intense, appropriate and simple.

Oriented means that our mind goes where we want it to go, so accidental stimuli do not disperse or quickly take it away. Acceptance implies that we encourage thoughts and feelings to come without opposition as various perceptions join and depart from our consciousness. We do not seek to evaluate or classify certain interactions as positive or poor. Lastly, simple means we have a vibrant and reliable understanding of what is happening, not a bland or ambiguous one.

Meditation allows us to respond to our discomfort by teaching these three values of concentration in a manner that minimizes our discomfort.

3. Regulating the response

Learning to pay heed to our suffering is a large aspect of the pain management plan. But we do need to be conscious of our reaction to pain. Aversion is one of our most normal and inevitable reactions to pain and we do not like it. We cannot easily turn off, but we can begin to realize it actively. When we are increasingly mindful of our reactions, we start managing or softening our very intense ones instinctively, allowing us to control our pain.

Here is how. Tune in to the suffering first. Then inquire of yourself, "when I feel this agony, what else occurs inside me?" You are not searching for a simple and fast solution. Rather, you direct your mind to the actual moment of your reaction to discomfort.

Occasionally, you might get a flood of troubled feelings, or primal anger. Some days it will be subtler or more shocking. I still remember when I first knew my suffering was making me feel healthy. I did not want to be in agony, but I felt terrified to live without it, as it had been so common over the decades. There is no longer a reason to react to your pain.

4. Putting the pieces together

An essential functional in meditation that can be used to deal with pain is called body scan. It is a process in which we gradually transfer our concentration to various areas of the body, beginning at the top of the head and moving downwards and back up once. Without analyzing or wanting to change anything we feel, we try to embrace and be responsive to any feelings encountered in the body.

If you feel unsure that the body scan exercise will work with your pain, note that mindfulness works with all types of pain irrespective of the cause. Practice responding to the stimuli in your body with the three virtues of attentive concentration, awareness, approval, and transparency. It takes time to build these attributes so be careful with yourself and continue. Eventually, ask yourself from time to time how you respond to the feelings in your body and spend a little time dreaming about what is coming up.

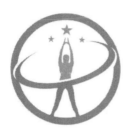

Chapter 11:
Science-Based
Benefits of Meditation

Meditation's success is growing as more people discover its advantages. Meditation is a repetitive method of preparing the mind to concentrate on the emotions and divert them. You do this experience consciousness of yourself and the environment. Some people think of it as a way to reduce anxiety and boost concentration. They use the exercise to build certain helpful behaviors and emotions, such as a good disposition and attitude, establish a life-discipline, enjoy a safe quality of sleep and even an improved acceptance of pain.

1. Reduces stress

Reducing stress is one of the main causes why people try meditation most often. One survey including more than 3,500 young people showed that meditation lives up to its reputation for relieving stress. Emotional and physical discomfort usually cause elevated levels of the cortisol stress hormone. This causes most of the adverse effects, like the discharge of inflammatory response-promoting neurotransmitters called cytokines. Such consequences can interfere with sleep, encourage stress and depression, raise blood pressure, and lead to tiredness and blurry thought.

In an eight-week analysis, the inflammatory reaction due to anxiety was minimized by a meditation style called "mindfulness meditation." Another survey of 1,300 young people showed that meditation can relieve stress. The influence was especially great in those with the maximum blood pressure. Research has revealed that meditation can also strengthen anxiety-related symptoms which include ulcerative colitis, fibromyalgia, and post-traumatic stress.

SUMMARY:

Multiple meditation forms encourage the lowering the tension. Meditation can also relieve pain of those in stress-induced health state.

2. Controls anxiety

Strong tension can turn into depression. For instance, an eight-week meditation analysis on mindfulness assisted participants in minimizing their depression. This decreased anxiety condition is seen in mental illnesses, social fear, intrusive feelings, neurotic-compulsive behaviors, and panic attacks. Further research followed up three years after 18 participants had finished an eight-week mediation program. Many participants had practiced daily exercise and retained reduced rates of deep anxiety.

A research study of 2,466 people similarly found that a range of meditation techniques could decrease anxiety levels. Yoga has been shown to assist people in controlling fear. This is attributed to gains both from meditative exercise and physical exercise. Meditation in elevated-pressure work settings can also assist in reducing job-related anxiety. One research study in fact showed a mediation system in a network of nurse's minimized anxiety.

SUMMARY:

Habitual therapy tends to minimize mental illnesses linked to fear and paranoia such as social pressure and neurotic-compulsive behavior phobia.

3. Promotes emotional health

A few types of meditation also contribute to a better self-image and a healthier perspective on life. Two therapy trials showed anxiety reduced in more than 4,600 people. One study followed 18 participants during three years of practicing meditation. The study showed long-term reductions in stress. Inflammatory neurotransmitters called cytokines produce stress that lead to depression and contribute to increased blood pressure. An analysis of many studies indicates therapy to reduce these inflammatory neurotransmitters may minimize stress. A further monitored research study measured electrical activity in the brains of individuals who performed meditation for consciousness compared to those of those who did not.

SUMMARY:

Some types of meditation can boost stress and make life more optimistic. Studies suggest that sustaining a continuing meditation practice will allow you to retain certain advantages long term.

4. Enhances self-awareness

Some types of meditation may assist you in building better self-understanding, enabling you to evolve into your true self. For starters, meditation on personality-inquiry is specifically meant to help you gain a deeper awareness of yourself and how you respond to those around you. Many types help you recognize the negative emotions that may cause you to lose yourself. The hope is that you will guide them into more positive behaviors as you develop a better understanding of your thinking process.

An analysis of 21 women battling breast cancer showed that their soul-esteem increased almost as much as it did in people who attended social therapy sessions. In another report, 40 senior men and women taking a meditation awareness plan experienced decreased in feelings of isolation relative to a test group on the program's waiting list. More innovative decision making can be promoted through the practice of meditation.

SUMMARY:

Soul-inquiry and similar mediation methods will help you "learn yourself." This may be a reference point for other meaningful improvements.

5. Lengthens attention span

Centered-attention exercise for better mental capacity is like powerlifting for the mind.. It boost your concentration power and stamina. For example, a research study investigated the impact of an eight-week course of meditation on mindfulness and showed it enhanced the capacity of learners to realign and retain their concentration. A related study found that human resources staff who frequently performed meditation on mindfulness remained focused on the job for way too long. Such staff have greater memory of the specifics of their activities compared to their colleagues who did not perform meditation.

In fact, one study revealed that meditation can also change brain processes that lead to mind roaming, anxiety and low concentration. You may also benefit from short periods of meditation. One study showed that four days of meditation practice could be necessary to improve mental capacity.

SUMMARY:

Various forms of meditation will develop the capacity to focus and hold awareness. It will have an impact in as little as four days.

6. May reduce age-related memory loss

Significant changes in mindfulness and depth of thought can help keep your mind healthy. Kirtan Kriya is a meditation technique that blends a mantra or chant with repeated finger movement to concentrate the mind. The increased capacity of subjects to execute memory tasks was seen in several trials on memory problems associated with age. In fact, a study of 12 experiments found that various meditation types in older participants enhanced concentration, memory, and neural speed.

In contrast to countering natural age-related memory damage, meditation in patients with dementia can at least to some extent boost memory. It may also help reduce depression and improve communication with other members of the family.

SUMMARY:

The increased concentration you can acquire from daily meditation will enhance attention and peace of mind. Both effects can help avoid the memory loss and depression associated with aging.

7. Can generate kindness

In fact, other kinds of meditation will generate optimistic emotions and behavior towards oneself and others. Metta is a form of meditation recognized as meditation on love-kindness; it helps to build kind thoughts and emotions towards oneself. Via practice people learn to apply compassion and acceptance, first to relatives, then to strangers, and eventually rivals.

Twenty-two studies of this kind of meditation have shown it's potential to raise the sympathy of people for themselves and others. One analysis of 100 adults chosen at random for a plan comprising mediation on caring-kindness found such effects to be stimulant-dependent. In other words, the more work people put into meditation on Metta, the more optimistic emotions they had. Another group of studies revealed that the optimistic emotions that people create from Metta mediation can increase social stress, decrease marital tensions, and control frustration. Such effects tend to grow over time with the application of meditation on love-kindness.

SUMMARY:

Metta, or meditation on caring kindness, is a method of cultivating optimistic emotions, first towards yourself and then towards others. Metta enhances optimistic mood, humility, and caring disposition towards others.

8. May help fight addictions

The mental strength you can build through meditation will help you break attachments by expanding self-control and acquiring knowledge of addictive habits. Studies have shown that meditation will assist people in focusing their energy, improving their resilience, regulating their feelings and desires, and strengthening their awareness of the reasons behind their addictive habits.

One research study that taught 19 alcoholics how to meditate found that people who learned the instruction were getting good at managing their anxieties and tension linked to cravings. Meditation in short helps manage food cravings. A summary of 14 studies showed that meditation in mindfulness helps to alleviate emotional and binge eating by participants.

SUMMARY:

Meditation improves strength of mind and determination, which can assist you to resist the undesirable thoughts that affect you. This will assist you to feel better, lose weight, and avoid certain unhealthy behaviors.

9. Improves sleep

By this point almost half the world is dealing with sleeplessness. One analysis contrasted two meditation systems and focused on mindfulness by choosing different participants for one of two classes. While one party performed mediation, the other did not. Participants who meditated slept early and remained longer unconscious, similar to those who did not meditate.

Being skilled in meditation will assist you in managing or diverting the racing or "runaway" mind, which often contributes to sleeplessness. It will also assist in calming your muscles, relieving anxiety and placing you in a relaxed state where you are more likely to fall asleep.

SUMMARY:

A variety of therapy methods can also assist you in calming and managing the "runaway" impulses that interrupt your sleep. This can reduce the time required to fall asleep and boost beneficial and normal sleep patterns.

10. Helps control pain

Your perspective of pain is linked to your mental state; and in stressful circumstances, it can be enhanced. For example, one research study used practical MRI methods to analyze brain activation when an unpleasant stimulus was felt by the participants. Few participants completed four days of mediation carefulness preparation and some did not. The meditating patients showed decreased activation in the center of the brain believed to regulate pain. They also registered comparatively less pain resistance.

With 3,500 participants, a broader study examined the impact of daily meditation. It considers meditation to be consistent with reduced chronic or occasional pain symptoms. Extensive meditation research on patients with advanced depression learned that it can alleviate severe end-of-life pain. Meditators and non-meditators faced the very exact sources of pain in both cases whereas meditators demonstrated a better capacity to deal with discomfort and also faced a decreased feeling of discomfort.

SUMMARY:

Meditation can reduce the sensation of mind pain. This can be used as an alternative to medical treatment or physiotherapy to relieve persistent pain.

11. Can decrease blood pressure

Meditation, too, will enhance cardiovascular health by minimizing heart stress. Over time, elevated blood pressure makes it difficult for the heart to supply enough blood, which can result in impaired cardiac function. Hypertension also leads to atherosclerosis, or artery shrinking, which can cause strokes and heart attacks. A survey of 996 participants in a study showed that meditating on a "silent mantra" — a repetitive, non-vocalized phrase — lowered blood pressure on by five figures.

This was particularly true for elderly participants and others who had elevated blood pressure before the test. An analysis found that identical changes in blood pressure resulted from many forms of meditation. In turn, meditation helps to regulate blood pressure by calming the nerve impulses that guide heart activity, blood vessel stiffness and the reaction of "fight-or-flight" that enhances alertness in tense situations.

SUMMARY:

In persons who meditate daily, blood pressure reduces not just during meditation but over time. This will lower stress on the heart and lungs and assist in avoiding heart disease.

12. You can meditate anywhere

People adopt several meditation methods, most of which need no specific tools or place. With only a few minutes of training, you can practice every day. If you really want to begin meditation, consider selecting meditation work based on what you want to obtain from it. There are two modes:

Oriented-attention meditation focuses attention on a specific object, including sound or the imagination. It focuses concentration by ridding any noise in your head. Meditation may be done with the breath, rhythm, or soothing tone.

Active-monitoring meditation promotes increased knowledge of all dimensions of the world through thought-training and self-sense. It can involve being conscious of emotions, desires, or urges that you may try to ignore. Seek the range of free, guided meditation activities and figure out which type you like the most. They are a perfect way to try various methods. If your daily working and home conditions do not afford secure, peaceful time alone, think about taking a class. Being part of a group culture will also increase your chances of success.

Try timing the alarm a couple of minutes early to get the benefit of morning quality time. This can assist you in creating a new routine and encourage you to have a productive day.

SUMMARY:

If you want to integrate meditation into your practice, check out a few different types and find supervised exercises for the one that suits you.

The Bottom Line

Meditation is something that everyone should use to enhance their physical and behavioral welfare. You can do it everywhere, without a services or membership. Optionally, there are freely accessible seminars on mediation and community groups. There is a wide range of approaches for differing abilities and desired effects. Try meditation to enhance your quality of life, and do it a few minutes every day.

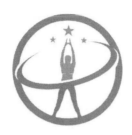

Chapter 12:
Ayurvedic Diet Plan: Get Rid of any Disease with One Diet

Ayurvedic Diet Plan

Would you like to avoid all illnesses in your life? Or do you have an illness and need to get relief naturally without medication? If yes, then this Ayurvedic diet plan should assist you in preventing sickness and getting relief.

Definition: The Ayurvedic diet is prescribed in Ayurveda to assist you in living a happy, healthful, and better life. The diet pattern is recognized as per Ayurvedic principles.

Such a plan fits everyone. Anybody can implement the Ayurvedic diet plan to accomplish their fitness goals or remain happier and more successful forever and live much longer lives.

Ayurvedic Diet Plan Principles

The main basic principles of the diet plan:

- Don't restrain hunger
- Only consume food when you are feeling actual appetite
- Consume two main meals per day – meal in the morning and meal in the evening
- Don't overconsume
- Consume the food in its natural form
- Consume food after forty-eight minutes of cooking. Do not store food for longer than three hours.
- Opt for home prepared meals
- Consume a meal with a calm mind

Ayurvedic Diet: Meal Timings

Nearly all classical Ayurvedic texts propose two main meals a day:

- Morning meal – three hours late after sunrise
- Evening meal – forty minutes exactly before sunset

Accordingly, the followings are good timings:

Meal Timings	During Long Days	During Short Days
Morning meal	8 am to 9 am	9 am to 10 am
Evening meal	5 pm to 6 pm	4 pm to 5 pm

What should I do if I feel appetite other than ay meal timings?

If it's not a false appetite, then you can consume the proper food from a main meal with a minimum of a two-hour gap. Among the healthful diets are:

- Fruits
- Fresh uncooked vegetables
- Fresh vegetable juice
- Coconut water

Those foods are easily digestible, nutrient-filled, and good for all people.

Ayurvedic Diet: Morning Meal

In fact, the morning meal should enjoyable. Your body needs energy all day long. So, in the morning you should be eating nutrient-rich food. Start taking fruit, whole grains, legumes (pulses), potatoes and yogurt.

Morning Food Ratio

Solid foods	1/2 part of the stomach
Water-rich foods	1/4 part of the stomach
Keep stomach empty	1/4 part of the stomach

Solid foods: Solid foods include seeds, lentils, whole grains, nuts and cooked vegetables.

Water-rich foods: Water-rich foods include fruits, apple juice, freshly squeezed juice, lemon water, soy milk, coconut water, etc.

Keep the stomach empty: You must eat just under your desire to eat forever. It implies leaving 1/4th of your stomach clean.

Morning Fruits

In the morning time, choose these fruits:

Apple	Pineapple	Plums	Guava
Grapes	Peaches	Cranberries	Orange
Apricots	Blackberry	Blue Berry	Pears
Dates	Figs	Grapefruit	Sweet Lime (Mosmi)
Cherries	Avocado	Berries	Prunes
Raspberry	Pomegranate	Sapodilla	

Restricted foods in the Morning

As per Yoga Ratnakar, avoid the following foods in the morning:

Mango	Banana	Dried ginger powder	Sesame
Chironji	Coconut Soup	Sugar Palm fruit	Gular (Cluster Fig Fruit)
Ankol	Jamun	Imli (Tamarind)	Ber (jujube)
Fresh amla fruits			

Ayurvedic Diet: Evening Meal

Evening Meal	Nutrient Dense

Food in the evening must be soft and laden with nutrients. You must eat fewer grains. You must also stop eating dead animals such as meat.

Evening Food Ratio

Solid foods	1/4 part of the stomach
Water-rich foods	1/2 part of the stomach
Keep stomach empty	1/4 part of the stomach

Solid Foods: Chapatis, rice, nuts, whole grains, seeds, and cooked vegetables are included in the category of solid foods.

Water-rich foods: Bananas, raw vegetables or salad, lime juice, coconut water or cow's milk (if accessible).

Keep stomach empty: 1/4th of the stomach must be empty.

Note: Do not consider tamarind water, amla water and amla milk on an empty stomach. Take them at night after a meal. After a meal, Ayurveda suggests these products.

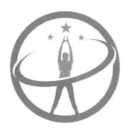

Conclusion

In yoga, the concept of purification is rife with great benefit. Individuals now connect spirituality with vegetarian food since it is non-violent to animals and indicates less blood toxicity. Similarly, spirituality is related to celibacy as it indicates lower body fluid pollution. Spirituality requires a safe and hygienic approach.

Yoga ideology is the consequence of human wisdom and experience in the realm of physiology, psychology, moral values as well as spirituality all gathered together for the well-being of mankind over hundreds of years.

The yogic way of managing stress is wholly holistic. The age-old practice of yoga has repeatedly proven its distinctiveness in relieving anxiety. It has been found that the impact of yoga is important for minimizing anxiety in women and in all aspects of life. There is every good reason to approach it for:

- the organizational area
- the family area
- the private area
- the area of social factors
- the area of external influences

Made in the USA
Middletown, DE
21 February 2022

61597316R00135